The Function

Modern Medicine for Modern Times

The Functional Medicine Handbook to Prevent and treat diseases at their root cause

Adonis Maiquez, M.D.

*"The doctor of the future will give no medicines,
but will interest his patients in the care
of the human frame, in diet,
and in the causes and prevention of disease."*
- Thomas A. Edison

ISBN-13: 978-1515260233
ISBN 10:1515260232

MEDICAL DISCLAIMER:
This book includes generalized information regarding medical illnesses and disease treatments. This is **not** given as medical advice and is for informational purposes only. Warranty is limited: The healthcare information provided within is furnished **without warranties**, stated or implied. The author and publisher make **no representations** as to information furnished in this book. Without prejudice to the previous paragraph, the author and publisher **do not** warrant that: the medical information herein is complete, true, accurate, up-to-date, or non-misleading.

Professional Assistance
Do not rely only on the information provided in this book, as a reason for not seeking medical advice. If you have any questions about your medical conditions consult your physician or health care professional immediately. Users accept full responsibility for seeking appropriate medical advice.

If you believe you have any condition, you should get medical care immediately. Never delay getting care from your physician, never disregard your physician's advice and do not discontinue medical treatment due to information in any book or website.

Liability
Nothing in this disclaimer is able to limit any of our liabilities in ways that are not permitted under the applicable law, or is able to exclude any liabilities that may not be excluded under the applicable law.

DEDICATION

I dedicate **MODERN MEDICINE for Modern Times** to every patient that I have had, over the last 25 years, who has entrusted me with their health and well-being and from whom I've learned so much.

By learning and following the modalities presented within, you can foresee a healthier life, with vitality, and longevity without the use of medications.

TABLE OF CONTENTS

PREFACE

The world is changing, and with it a new form of medicine, for these modern times is needed. I believe in a shift from acute care and medication-based to evaluating and addressing the underlying causes of health care issues as a new model of treatment; Modern Medicine for these Modern Times.

Modern times truly do require modern medicine. Our 21st century life has brought about untold challenges including environmental pollution, soil nutrient deprivation, babies being born with toxicities and immune systems that are weak, the effects of radiation of all types that we aren't aware of, and the overuse of antibiotics that destroy the normal healthy intestinal flora, just to name a few issues.

In reality it's almost as if a "new human" or a mutated form of who we used to be has been created. These changes create diseases that cannot be treated with the current healthcare approach of using yet another chemical (pharmaceutical medications).

What we need to do is to get to the root cause of these problems and try to re-balance our bodies back to their original state. It's like rebooting the body to the state that nature has intended. This book is a paradigm shift in medicine. MODERN MEDICINE for these modern times is a shift that is needed to solve humanity's current chronic disease epidemic.

Today's healthcare and treatment model doesn't really allow for the necessary time that your doctor needs to consider the entirety of you as a human being, and discovering exactly what is behind one or more symptoms you are feeling.

We'll get into the time-shortage reasons later, but suffice it to say that we human beings are integrated organisms made up of a complex set of systems, which operate in an integrated manner so that we can go about our daily lives, whether we are working, playing, sleeping, eating or doing any of the many thousands of things that active humans do.

When the human being is out of sync, things go wrong, people get sick, sometimes they get chronically ill, and often some calamity occurs and they are thrown into a healthcare system that would scare the heck out of anyone seeing it for the first time.

Today's methods are a bit limited. Usually:

1.   You will bring the doctor a short list of your symptoms
2.   The doctor does a cursory exam, part of it is done by nurses, (vital signs, weight, height, etc.)
3.   The doctor then palpates and/or checks you for the symptoms if at all (thorough physical exams are rarely done these days)
4.   The doctor either requests tests (blood, urine, stool, X-rays, scans etc.) or
5.   From your medical history and his years of experience with research, education, studies of treatments of the symptoms, takes out his little white pad, writes you a prescription for some chemically-produced pharmaceutical medication to make the symptom more tolerable, or make the symptom completely go away, at least temporarily.

But the symptom treated isn't really gone. What's really happening is that it's burrowing underground, deeper within the same bodily system, whether digestive, respiratory, circulatory, etc. The symptom may be gone temporarily, but for example, gastritis treated by a prescription might actually transform into stomach cancer.

Although this might happen as an end game resulting from not treating the person as a whole, other symptoms may occur within the same system and another prescription may be given for the new symptom. Then the chemicals mix together in the stomach and there is certainly the potential for the chemicals to damage the stomach, the intestines, and other systems throughout the body.

It's far wiser to gain the knowledge of what caused the primary symptom, and use the modalities presented herein to you, which are derived from the field of Functional Medicine to clean out any irritant or toxin from your body, build your immunity, and let your body heal itself naturally.

It's Your Choice

The methods of care and treatment, and who your doctor is that works with you, towards achieving your own level of health and balance in life is all a matter of choice. You can select from many branches of medicine and healthcare, and whichever branch you choose, I hope that your chosen physician has studied the field of Functional Medicine to help your entire body, and the modalities presented that will help you return to optimum health that we will shortly discuss.

To give you a reason, let me begin by saying that I am a medical doctor who works with a specialty in Functional Medicine. Too often we get patients who have problems with their thyroid glands and the cause is an autoimmunity disorder. Simply stated, these patients usually say that they have a problem going on and don't know exactly what it is.

> *Apparently, there's now a well-documented connection between those with illnesses that have been treated by pharmaceutical medication for long periods of time, and the symptoms still prevail, and doctors and the pharmaceutical industry are looking for other answers. You'll find those answers here in this book.*

This is because the doctor they've chosen to supervise, and evaluate the symptom, might do only one test (allowed by the insurance company) and give a prescription for medication for the patient's diagnosed symptom, which may or may not help. Perhaps later, they will try a second or third medication over a period of time – but in reality, it will not really discover or treat the systemic problem which caused the disease because it has never been diagnosed, nor have they found the root causes of it.

But, the undiagnosed problem could have been helped another way. Had the physician looked at the whole person, rather than one symptom, the process would have been easier, faster, and more complete – and the natural healthful state would return and last for the entirety of the life of the patient.

As a physician, I can tell you, that learning about your symptoms can tell me a great deal about your health, but treating you by eliminating symptoms with medication, rather than checking for possible links between a variety of symptoms and a variety of bodily systems, is not the smartest way of attaining total and complete bodily health. Treating only the patient's symptoms, with medication, may not have much success.

I know how important each of the different bodily systems are to the health of your whole body and how important it is to look at the whole person, their whole body when treating them, as a physician. I have followed the Functional Medicine approach to finding the connections for every patient I see from the beginning of my work with them.

Life is influenced by many factors. All of human existence is influenced as well. Nothing in life is ever solely caused by one factor. There seems to be some form of interrelation between all elements and all of the processes in life. The factors seem to be working together all the time, mostly 9 operating in unison.

As an example: a wildflower growing in the woods doesn't get water one day, sunlight exposure the next day, and then on another day soil nutrients. The flower gets all that it needs simultaneously as nature provides it through a process that is similar to drip irrigation - whereby water, sunlight, and nutrients are received in a trickle-down process. That's what nature provides and intended to obviously attain the best results for accomplishing natural flower growth.

In my experience as a Functional Medicine practitioner, the best results are accomplished through nine areas of life which I've identified over the last 12 years, while treating patients, especially those with chronic health issues.

When all of these specific protocols are managed together using Functional Medicine modalities, it considerably diminishes any potential of reoccurring health issues.

So, from the outset, let's make this perfectly clear. this book is NOT about using any one fix, or one discovery. This book is about the knowledge, which I have personally accumulated from helping patients to regain their optimum health, and stay healthy. In front of you, is a protocol – one that will make sense for your health and well-being every day of your life.

Thousands of Guidebooks – In the Wrong Direction

There are thousands of books written on hundreds of different aspects of improving your health. Some are right on, and others are just a bit of hocus pocus. As with other concepts of medicine and healthcare, the major issue with these books is that they don't really address YOU as a whole being, as an individual, as an entity, as an integrated unit of many operating systems. And that integrated unit is influenced by many aspects including your birth family genetics, your medical history, your lifestyle, your diet, and the environment in which you live.

More than that, this book contains a protocol or a system that you can use to better your health and life. You might also realize that it includes a great deal of scientific information, which I have attempted to simplify, so you realize how science has played a huge role in proving that this protocol is science-based and will work for you. At any time, if you feel the concepts are too complex to understand, just skip reading them, and move on to the next section. You can always go back and read the scientific research or evidence at a later time if you feel the need to do so.

The book was written in this way so that you could learn the protocol, and have the backup scientific data should you ever need to explain it to others.

Balance is What We Seek

We all know that nature is about equilibrium. No matter what goes on in the world, that impacts nature – nature will survive and regain its balance. That is not what happens with our human bodily systems, until we reach that point of living more in balance and harmony with the natural protocol in Functional Medicine.

Homeostasis

As I said earlier, nature is all about balance. Nature has been around for billions of years, and no matter what occurs on the surface of earth, hurricanes, tornados, volcanos, etc., nature seeks out and finds ways, over time, to recreate a sense of balance.

Now, wouldn't it be great if your body could react in the same way and over time it recreated that sense of balance, healthfulness, proper weight for your height and frame. Having your body do whatever you need it to do – whether it is having an active family life with your children, or being an athlete performing at your best, or even living a fashionable life - dressed to a T, looking great at the parties you attend, on your way up the corporate or social ladder. That would be a blessing.

Balance is achievable. But, it takes some work to get started having Functional Medicine work for you the way you want. So, let's get to work on it.

The Need for a New Medicine

Modern times, with its Agricultural, Industrial and Information Revolutions, have brought great advances to our lifestyle and comfort. But it has also created the landscape for harmful effects on our health. Especially over the last 100 years we have seen a rapidly increasing ill effect on our health from the following:

- Environmental toxins from factories, automobiles, and other sources contaminating the water supply, air, and soil

- Radiation from cell phones, cell phone towers, and microwaves
- Soil nutrient content deprivation
- Food preparation techniques to improve preservation that destroy enzymes and nutrients
- Overuse of steroids, antibiotics, and hormones on livestock.
- Overprescribing of antibiotics for people, which has created "super bugs" and destroyed the normal healthy intestinal (bacterial) flora
- Overuse of anti-depressants, attention deficit disorders, and other psych meds that are even finding their ways to water sources and the soil
- Poly-pharmacy (the use of multiple prescription and over the-counter drugs)
- A more stressed society where the media is in constant "alert"
- A shortened attention span with people being less able to meditate and contemplate
- Increased addiction rates not only to chemicals but to technology
- Excessive use of food preservatives, colorants, and artificial sweeteners
- Lack of physical activities due to the availability of motorized transportation means and elevators

All these factors have created a unique environment for many chronic "modern diseases" to escalate. Diseases that were rare before, are now a lot more common and new diseases are developing all the time.

Over the last few years there has been a sharp increase in:
- Cancers
- Autoimmune diseases (like lupus, MS, arthritis, Grave's)
- Diabetes, obesity, and metabolic syndrome
- Cardio-vascular diseases (high blood pressure, heart

disease, and stroke)
- Mental diseases like depression, anxiety, addictions, social isolation
- Neurological diseases (Alzheimer's dementia, Parkinson's, ADD, autism)
- Chronic respiratory diseases like asthma, COPD, emphysema
- Allergies, skin, and respiratory
- Chronic or persistent infections (viruses like HIV, CMV, EBV) (bacterial like Rocky Mountain Fever) (candida)
- Hormone imbalances
- Diseases that are difficult to classify like fibromyalgia, chronic fatigue, non-specific mental fogginess

So, there is an obvious need for a different approach. The already existing old approach of "pill medicine" giving a medication for every symptom is not working anymore. This approach might be creating even more problems than solutions, which I will discuss in this book. The solution I recommend is to address the actual root causes of the problem, not the end-result complaint or symptoms, but what is causing it. We should not look for an isolated "target" to go after, but look at the individual at their foundation - and look at them as a whole, physical, mental, and spiritual unity while trying to recover that lost balance or homeostasis.

A Word About Prevention

The recommendations and protocols presented in this book (and other books of this Series) apply not only to the amelioration or resolution of diseases already in place but to the prevention of those diseases as well. It is my experience in my clinical practice that when people apply these concepts and address health at the root cause, the onset of certain diseases (even when there is a genetic predisposition) can be delayed.

Even if you have a strong family history of diabetes, Alzheimer's, heart disease or any other chronic disease, the development of that disease can be postponed and even aborted completely. This can only be accomplished when you modify the foundations of what causes the disease in the first place.

"Early screening" does not prevent disease. It merely detects it at an early stage so it is easier to treat. The real benefit lies in preventing or delaying the appearance of the disease, avoiding much suffering, disability, and healthcare expenses.

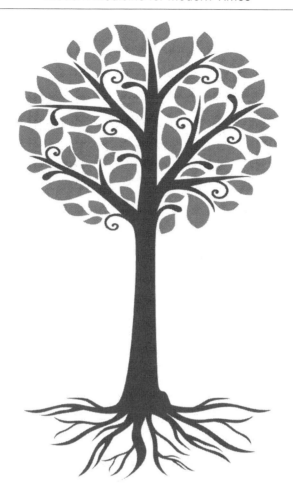

ACKNOWLEDGMENTS

I want to express my sincerest thanks:

To my parents, for believing in me, no matter what the circumstances were during my life. Please accept my thanks for all your support.

To my siblings, for supporting me, and sometimes literally doing so, so that I might continue to pursue my career, while having food on the table.

To my daughter, Maia Sophia, who has brought a higher level of inspiration to my daily life.

To my wife, Luly, for her unconditional love and care when I was busy with my work and writing this book, when I should have been with her, relaxing and enjoying our lives together.

To Dr. Jay Polmar and Maria Krebs for improving the text and giving it structure.

To Maria Krebs and Cecilia Gonzalez Garcia for translating and editing the Spanish version.

To Lili Gonzalez Garcia and Martha Garcia Marquez for the design and layout of the various versions of this book.

I want to thank and acknowledge all of you for helping create the homeostasis, and just the right balance of pressure and encouragement, to bring this work to fruition.

A special thanks to my staff, past and present, who have always treated me and our patients, with so much respect and care: THANK YOU!!!

How to use this book in your daily life

Imagine that you are in a classroom, and you are studying human biology and this particular class is aimed at improving personal health, and living a life of being fit and healthy all the time.

That is how it has been designed and written to give you the scientific data and the 'straight facts' on how your body works and what you need to do to have your body work all the time, functioning perfectly for a long and healthy life.

Once you finish the course, there is a final exam. That final exam is putting the course into use and getting an A is based on your condition of healthfulness and being fit.

When some of the scientific data is just too much to take in, mark the pages you did not read inside the front cover, and when you feel it is time to study those more difficult concepts, go back and read or re-read them. The result of the course will be the same whether or not you understand the difficult concepts.

"The doctor of the future —
will give no medicine, but —
will interest his patients in the
care of the human body,
in diet, and in the cause
and prevention of disease."

- Thomas A. Edison

INTRODUCTION TO FUNCTIONAL MEDICINE

After reviewing the history of medicine, I'd like to think that Functional Medicine is a "returning to the body" of medical sciences. Medicine used to focus on body, mind, and spirit - as a whole, and especially on the interrelation of all elements or components, including the surrounding environment and its impact on health. It was like that for thousands of years.

Now, during "modern" times, healthcare has focused on pharmaceuticals and chemicals to treat specific complaints, or measurements (blood pressure, blood sugar just to mention a few) without looking at the individual, as a whole entity, with all our parts or components being intimately related and impacting each other.

Functional Medicine starts from the point that health becomes attainable when all the elements that make up the whole are in perfect harmony. The same complaint (headache, heartburn, fatigue, high blood pressure) may have been caused by a myriad of malfunctions throughout a chain of elements in the entire system.

So, if you address only one of the areas (for example taking an anti-inflammatory pill for joint pain) without addressing the baseline issues (which might be a food sensitivity which causes an autoimmune complex formation that deposits on the joints, or a vitamin deficiency that needs supplementation for the natural auto-inflammatory enzyme reactions in the joints), this will not address the root causes. So, the treatment will only be temporary and usually will have side effects from the medications.

Complaints and symptoms begin many years before they become obvious enough to become named as a "disease." Modern physicians have been effective in grouping those symptoms and naming diseases (i.e. Parkinson's, Alzheimer's, and many others). But they have not been effective in dealing with these complaints when they first begin, many years before symptoms turn into a "full blown" disease.

Functional Medicine tries to address the imbalances when they first occur. Many chronic diseases have common starting points (inflammation, oxidation, food sensitivities, immune dysregulation, etc.) that when addressed at onset can halt or delay the appearance of an end-stage disease. By concept, Functional Medicine is patient based (individualized medicine) and not disease based (when a diagnosis or disease becomes made and named, then all treatment is the same for all people thus affected).

The clinical thinking process of Functional Medicine is not conceptually different from that of modern Western medicine but it differs in its approach. It is still comprised of reviewing how the person got to the current point (medical history), examining the body looking for clues (physical exam), investigating with laboratory and diagnostic tests (diagnostics) and recommending actions to take to change the current and future health and wellbeing (treatment or therapeutics).

Medical History:

A medical history is obtained, but it goes back predating conception, pregnancy, childhood and recent events, and how they all affect health. Most of the time when the initial insult is found (for example a major trauma) in the past, the current symptoms trace back to how that event affected the immune or hormonal systems. Any prior abuse of antibiotics (so prevalent today) can give a glimpse of the person's intestinal flora, which in turn determines gut permeability and ultimately the development of autoimmune diseases.

This is most important for treatment decision making, because an "autoimmune" disease like rheumatoid arthritis sometimes should not be treated with immune-modulators (which have major side effects), but with food elimination, probiotics, and gut restoration (we will discuss this later in the book).

Physical Exam:

Most patients complain that modern doctors do not "touch" their patients anymore. Even though modern medicine was originally based on an exhaustive examination of the patient (and even tasting of their urine by the doctor), the most recent medical model has distanced the doctor from the patient's human body. Physical examination has become replaced by machines.

A doctor trusts more in a CT scan than his stethoscope. Since Functional Medicine emphasizes prevention and early intervention, a comprehensive physical exam is mandatory. The functioning of the organs and systems cannot be detected by machines, only obvious anatomical changes can. The interconnection between all the bodily systems, the harmony of the body, with the mind and the spirit, can only become assessed by talking to and examining the patient.

Diagnosis:

Even though the taking of a thorough medical history and a physical exam might be all that's needed to determine where the imbalances are, the diagnostic or "detective" aspect of medicine still has an important role in Functional Medicine. Sometimes diagnostictests are needed to determine which elements, pillars, or "key supports" are altered. Even when one of them is functioning properly the interrelation between all of them is not.

Those key supports (see the chapter on supports) and the harmonious interaction between them are why a patient has a healthy body, mind, and spirit.

The goal of the Functional Medicine practitioner is to identify those supports and determine which one, or which ones, or which pathways between them changed or became imbalanced, and correct that issue. Also, the human body is "wired" in such a way that it is capable of healing itself, and most of the time all that needs to be done is to remove the obstacles that are in the way of that self- healing or natural self-renewal process.

Treatment or Therapeutic Recommendations:

Like I said before, treatment in Functional Medicine sometimes involves minimal intervention. Sometimes, it is as simple as removing the obstacles to self-healing. However, other times, there are many areas affected and an intervention is required. This is accomplished by using several principles that address the foundation of the body functions. The main actions that the physician performs are:

- Adjust (eliminate or include) the foods consumed according to the person's genetic composition and his or her previous food exposure. Besides the recommendations for everybody - to avoid certain types of food (mainly large amount of sugars, grains - especially wheat, toxic food additives, and sweeteners) most people have developed sensitivities to specific foods during their lifetime. Eliminating them, usually only temporarily, gives the body a "break" from the effect of the wrong food. Incorporating certain foods which have healing properties (like some herbs) will also speed up recovery, and allow the person to regain homeostasis or balance.

- Replenish the elements that might be deficient and aren't needed for normal physiologic bodily functions, like vitamins and nutrients. All bodily functions not only need energy sources (proteins, fats or carbohydrates) but also need minerals and vitamins that make possible all its functions. Not only does a lack of energy sources cause a weakened system, but also a deficiency of those "facilitators" can cause disease. Several scientific studies have shown that sometimes, simply taking a specific vitamin, can result in the decrease of chances of acquiring certain diseases (for example, there is a link between vitamin D deficiency and depression or cancer).

- Eliminating undesired toxins from the body that might be impairing the normal performance of the body's functions. These can include heavy metals (mercury, aluminum, and others), preservatives (paraben), organo-phosphates in insecticides and herbicides, petrochemical derivatives used to manufacture plastics, rubber and dyes, to mention just a few. Detoxification is an ongoing process we all must endure in the polluted modern day environment we live and work in. Daily detoxification is one of the most useful tools to preserve and recover health today. Later, in this book, I will give recommendations on how to do just that.

> **Prescription medications are not rejected by Functional Medicine. Modern Pharmacology has made a tremendous contribution especially in antibiotic therapies for infections that used to wipe out entire populations.**

- Prescription medications have a place in the methodology of the functional practitioner. A most important aspect of today's medicine is not only to over-prescribe medications, but to remove the side effects of those. Most prescription medications produce changes in the normal functioning of the body's processes, which in turn create nutritional deficiencies that can affect other functions. See references at the end of the book to become aware of which nutrients need to become replaced when taking specific medications.

- Body, Mind, and Spirit: It is not by coincidence that meditation was (and is) an important part of Ayurvedic medicine. Mindfulness is even recognized by modern Psychology as an important aspect of mental health.

One of the most devastating mistakes of modern medicine is that it forgot the interconnectedness between all the elements that compose the whole and how they interact with each other to attain balance. Each microscopic and macroscopic part of the body is interconnected with each other. From the cell in the intestine to the neuron in the brain, from the food antigen to the knee joint, from the brain's neurotransmitter to the stomach being satisfied, there is a connection.

Moreover, all of these anatomic and physiologic parts, that interconnect, are closely related to the mind and spirit. Health is nothing more than a perfect balance of our physical, emotional, and spiritual bodies inside us, interconnected with others, the world, and the Universe.

CHAPTER ONE
The History of Medicine

ANCIENT MEDICINE

While discovering edible plants, Stone Age humans discovered that some of those plants could cure ailments. Herbs in medicinal treatments began in the earliest days of medical treatment and remain today, in many countries, as a vital part of medical treatment.

Herbal medicines were but a tiny portion of the repertory of the tribal medicine man/physician, because it had always been generally accepted, except for modern day allopathic medicine, that serious illnesses have a spiritual causation. Back then, it was the tribal doctor's responsibility to expel evil spirits that were at the cause of the trouble. Incantations, spells, and trances often induced by herbal medicines formed the work of medicine men or shamans. Even the earliest operation, over 4,000 years ago, was probably intended to strengthen the doctor in some way; at least in the eyes of others.

It appears that the earliest surgeries in human history were carried out in prehistory throughout Asia and Europe. In Peru, as well, carefully preserved mummified bodies survived the passage of time. Many of these mummified human beings have a hole in the skull from trepanning (a surgical procedure where a hole is drilled and/or scraped into the human skull, to expose the dura mater to treat problems stemming from intracranial diseases), which as many as 50 percent survived.

It is speculated that the reasoning behind the decision to make a hole in the head of a live person had some religious or spiritual purpose rather than a medical purpose. Being a survivor of that type of surgery, the shaman has proven to the tribe that he is favored by the spirit world. A surgery to the skull, once it was healed, suggested an unseen open channel of spiritual communication with the supernatural.

SHAMANIC MEDICINE

Shamanism

Shamanism is deeply connected to nature. It is one of the most ancient forms where people have sought a link to the powers and origins of creation. It dates as far back as the Paleolithic times. Aspects of shamanism were reflected in many later religions, often in their symbolic and mystic rituals. Shamanism influenced Greek paganism. Several shamanic rituals common to the religion adopted by the Greeks were afterward seen also in the religion of the Romans. The shamans left their mark on the Bon religion which stems from central Asia, as well as in Buddhism and Tibetan Buddhist history.

Buddhism was popularized through shamanic groups like the Mongols, Tibetans, and Manchu. Various types of shamanistic practices merged into Tibetan Buddhism transformed the Tibetan religion in the time of the Chinese Yuan dynasty; later into the Qing dynasty. A commonality between the shamans and the Buddhists is demonstrated in their goal of spiritual awareness, sometimes assisted through the use of psychedelics. Shamanic rituals of various populations were almost entirely destroyed, due to the growth of Christianity.

In Europe, beginning in around 400 AD, the Catholic Church started destroying Greek and Roman religions. Temples were demolished and religious rites became illegal and punishable. Continuing into the Renaissance, the remainder of European shamanism was eradicated by witch hunts. These were often conducted by the Catholic Inquisition. Priests of the Catholic church were often instrumental in destroying local beliefs and rituals, in South America, Central America, and parts of the Caribbean. In some areas of Latin America, priests were beheaded for interfering with shamans.

In North America, the Puritans campaigned against "witches." Attacks on shamans were orchestrated by Christian missionaries in third-world countries. As recently as the 1970s, ancient rock drawings in the Amazon were ruined by missionaries. Today, shamanism survives for the most part only among various isolated indigenous peoples, and strongly in South America. Shamanic religion continues in the deserts, jungles, tundras, and other remote locations, also in some cities, small towns, even in suburbs and out to shantytowns around the world.

Many efforts have been made to connect Western scientific beliefs with shamanic practice. Jeremy Narby, a renowned anthropologist, believed shamans utilized their consciousness at the molecular level, and perhaps even worked with viruses and DNA. David Bohm's Holomovement theory is often viewed as some type of attempt to create a scientific foundation for concepts in spirituality including parallel worlds.

Many women have been vitally important in the shamanic field worldwide, and in some cultures, they are more important than others. This was exemplified in ancient Japan and China, and it still appears to be the same in Korea today as well with tribes in South Africa, and also with the Yuroks and Karoks in northern California. Images, traditions, and history show women as invokers, healers, herbalists, oracles, shape shifters, shamanic journeyers, and priestesses of the ancestors.

Some burials of females in ancient Central Asia were proclaimed by archeologists to be shamanic priestesses. A priestess from the Ukoks (5th century BCE) was entombed with a framed headdress that was decorated with a symbol of the Tree of Life. Similar burials were found at Ussun' (Kazakhstan), and also nearby in the Ukraine, with reappearing themes of medicine bags, incense, amulets, and the Tree of Life.

Invocatory chants are still an integral part of Mexican Indian shamanism. Chanting and then shaking of a rattle considered highly sacred were a part of the rituals of Katjambia, a medicine woman in the Himba tribe, residing in Namibia. After taking the energies that are negative into her, Katjambia then uses them as vision to return into the sacred fire of her ancestors, and they then release the energies for her.

The power of healing practiced by many female shamans was often described as restoring life to the dead. Pa Sini Jobu, the Tungutu of Niger's Bosso people, danced himself to ecstasy, and turned into a great bird, echoing the tales of the god Isis. In western Africa, sorceress Kulutugubaga heals as well as brings the dead to life.

Spanish and Portuguese colonials punished female Filipino shamans, naming them "devil-ridden old women" and "witches." Mayan oracles as well as shamans were faced with the same. The conquering Spanish imposed their ideas on Peruvian shamans, especially using the theme of the devil.

The Healers & Witches

The archetype of the healer is old and interesting. Every culture from the earliest peoples through to modernity has had some sort of healer in their culture. It is a part of life to be hurt, whether physical, emotional, or spiritual. Because of this, there has always been someone who is ready and able to help the injured.

For many peoples who had little understanding of the body and how it worked, healing seemed like magic. There are still mysteries around healing. In Native American culture the shamans believed they could communicate with the spirit world in the form of animals to help them in their healing work.

Witches were healers, especially in pagan beliefs where worship of nature came naturally for healers. The image of the witch stirring her potions, and mixing dry herbs and powdered materials together with mortar and pestle gave the healer a negative image for hundreds of years. Witches were tortured and killed for their healing, which was called devilish. However, female healers were often the only people peasants could turn to for medical help. The midwife is a good example of an enlightened healing figure; she supports the mother, who does the actual physical work of birth.

Many monks were learned in plants and herbs and practiced healing themselves. Priests would lay their hands on the sick and be called upon as well to perform last rites over the dead and dying.

By the 1800s the country doctor making house calls was a common sight. Midwifery was a branch of medicine also, but it had to be kept underground. Midwives did more than deliver babies and many were as knowledgeable and talented as the male doctors, or more so. Eventually, women became more involved in treating patients and at some point, started becoming surgeons.

Modernized Practices

After WWI, practices changed and hospitals became more like businesses. Medicine began being practiced in offices and clinics and certain educational degrees were now needed to practice. Drugs entered the field; science and medicine had finally begun to meet. Doctors learned to diagnose conditions and dispense medicines. However, holistic medicine was becoming more and more popular. Alternative medicine included practices like homeopathy, acupuncture, herbalism, and others. There were also treatments which targeted both physical and emotional health such as Reiki, Quantum-Touch therapy, therapeutic massage, aromatherapy, kinesiology, and yoga.

HINDU MEDICINE

The Buddha, born in India around 450 AD, created the teachings that form the basis of the Buddhist tradition. These teachings, from the Nikāyas or Āgamas texts, concern the finding of liberation from suffering. The ultimate goal of Buddha's teachings is to help us attain the good life. His view is that the source of suffering involves claims concerning human nature, as well as how we learn about our world and our place in this world.

Susruta, the founder of Hindu medicine, established a tradition, later written about in the Susruta Samhita, which named 1120 diseases and listed 760 drugs. It was said the equipment of their surgeons included about 20 sharp tools (including needles, scissors, knives, and saws) and over 100 blunt instruments (including hooks, tubes, forceps, levers, and probes). His conceptualizations included descriptions of blood tissue, our circulatory process (he called that rakta dhatu) and his research into the therapeutic value of minerals which were specially treated that he called bhasmas. He was given the title of father of iatrochemistry. His description of his method of rebuilding a damaged nose gave him the title of the world's first plastic surgeon.

Medicine in early India follows an idea that the body is made of a trio of substances, (spirit, phlegm, and bile), and proper health needs a balance of these humors. Greek medicine advanced a similar theory, based on four humors. Shortly after that came Ayurvedic Medicine, brought by Nagarjuna, who was also born in India and a disciple of Buddha. He is considered the most important philosopher after Buddha, who was an Ayurveda practitioner.

AYURVEDIC MEDICINE

Ayurveda: Philosophy and History

Ayurveda is based on an ancient way of understanding (ayur means knowledge and veda means life). It began in India centuries ago from a profound belief in and understanding of how creation occurred. The visionaries of ancient India understood it by meditating and using other spirituality. They attempted to spread the truths of physiology and health through the ages. They had spent great periods of time observing the fundamentals of life and thus, they compiled India's texts of philosophy and spiritual truth into books called the ***Bhagavad Gita***, the Veda of Knowledge.

The first publications of Ayurveda were the Veda and they remain among the world's oldest writings that exist today. There are three vital texts of the Veda, which are believed to be over 1,200 years old. These books are still being used today throughout the world. At first, this knowledge was passed down from the teacher to the student by mouth only, and was not written down until later.

Ayurveda inspired many health clinicians both in the West and East. By the beginning of the 5th century AD, Ayurvedic writings had been transcribed by the Chinese. By the early 8th century AD, scholars from China began studying medicine in India. Quickly, Chinese medicine was affected, and so was the Buddhist philosophy. Today, Ayurveda is essentially the same way it was in the beginning.

Ayurveda is a teaching of conceptual systems which is depicted by balance and disorder. Health and disease, according to Ayurveda, are regulated by our connection between our self (soul), our personality, and all events within our mental, spiritual, and spiritual beings. To maintain good health, a harmonic balance (later labeled by Hans Selye, MD as homeostasis), must exist. To gain that homeostasis, there is a balance that can be achieved through a combination of yoga, Buddhism, and Ayurvedic. Yoga is Ayurveda's sister science. They are born from the same philosophy.

Ayurveda is a meticulous mixture of several Hindu philosophical systems, many behavioral and physical sciences, and their combined medical practices. Ayurvedic medicine aims to heal existing conditions, to maintain health, and to prevent disease. Health may be called the feeling of happiness or a sense of bliss in the mind, the soul and the senses. Its central principle states human life is an integration of body, mind, senses, and spirit. Ayurveda believes that nothing would exist without a supreme consciousness that they believe to be all powerful and all knowing, a pervasive spirit and life force which expresses through creation. Ayurveda seeks the knowledge of this level of life.

Ayurveda requires that the function of creation be understood in the exchange of three elemental energy complexes, Vata, Pitta and Kapha — which signify dynamic, energetic, non-material aspects of nature; the intellect, the transformative nature, and the human structural, which is physical nature.

Vata governs:
- respiration
- circulation
- elimination
- movement
- speech
- creativity
- enthusiasm

- the nervous system

Pitta includes transformations such as:
- digestion and metabolism
- vision, complexion
- body temperature
- courage
- cheerfulness
- intellect
- discrimination

Kapha governs:
- growth (anabolic processes)
- lubrication
- fluid secretions
- binding
- potency
- patience
- heaviness
- fluid balance
- compassion
- understanding in the organism

These three Ayurvedically explained energies express themselves in the human body. It is called Tridosha. The total of these 3 Doshas - Kapha, Pitta, and Vata, orchestrate a person's physical and functions, which include the metabolism and the mind/body type.

These energies are meant to interact in a balanced manner. Their expression in the human being, indicates a ratio of these energies by one's DNA (Vata-Pitta-Kapha ratio), established in each human at the time of conception. This is called Prakruti, or constitutional typing.

Seven types of Prakruti exist:
- Vata
- Pitta
- Kapha
- plus four combinations thereof

Prakruti gives us two vital understandings:
- First, every person has a perpetual nature for their full term of life.
- Second, each type shows an area most likely to go out of harmony, requiring lifelong care.

The implication in medicine indicates that we have a natural tendency toward some medicines. Imbalance takes place because an energy or element is increased or altered qualitatively. Because these three governing ideologies are energy themselves, they tend to affect either opposite or similar energies. Pitta is intensified by heat, Vata is intensified by dryness, and Kapha is intensified by liquid.

Therefore, an upset in the balance of these energies indicates that something has stimulated and overpowered the ability of the human body to maintain Prakruti or balance in the ratio of Vata-Pitta-Kapha. If the system and the stimulus contain a similar or the same energy, the stimulation causes an increase of itself. This can create an imbalance even when the energies are not really unhealthy alone.

For example, well-prepared organic dishes can still cause imbalance when eaten in excess or at incorrect times. Over time, chronic conditions, and some defects in the body (caused by genes, disease, trauma, congenital defect, or other pre-existing conditions), cause disease to develop in a weak organ or tissue.

Ayurvedic medicine has three types of treatments.
These broad groups include:

- elimination treatment (shodana or panchakarma) Ayu
- pacification treatment (shamana)
- nourishing treatment (bhrimana)

Panchakarma is comprised of:
- nasal administration for Vata, Pitta, and Kapha
- medicated enemas for Vata
- bloodletting for Pitta
- vomiting for Kapha

Ayurvedic medication believes, as does Functional Medicine, that symptomatic treatment is ineffective in curing a disease. Some pacification therapies, which are balancing through the use of opposites, include:
- diet
- lifestyle
- herbs
- meditation
- yoga
- and more

Treatments to nourish are utilized for issues of physical power or strength to be treated. A classic Ayurveda development of disease is described in six steps. Knowing the symptoms of each step, for every dosha helps the doctor who has studied Ayurvedic medicine to diagnose and treat. For example, this wisdom thus demonstrates how a cold may become asthma or turn into congestive heart failure.

In Ayurvedic philosophy, creation consists of the five elements: ether, air, fire, water, and earth. This is how Ayurvedic healing works. When those elements are resilient and in harmony, they maintain a healthy body function. Illnesses are viewed as dosha aggravations to the human body. A doctor who has studied Ayurvedic medicine will determine what part of their patient's life has created an imbalance, whether it is dietary, lifestyle, work, or emotions, etc.

For measurable dosha changes, such as gas, hormones, and mucus, therapies of elimination (Panchakarma) are utilized. For qualitative changes, taking care of localized issues, like a sprain or strain, are managed through application of opposites (pacification) through diet, by making lifestyle changes, and through the use of herbal medications, etc. Pacification's role is to make subordinate the therapies of elimination involved in Panchakarma, but physiological balance must be achieved in the end. When the problem is toxicity, detoxification and digestive herbs are put to good use. Mental and spiritual disorders of the mind require specific treatment for the mind and spiritual. These could involve mantras, rituals, and other spiritual elements.

The study of Ayurveda is comprehensive and takes time; its Pharmacopeia is huge. At its central premise is the belief that no disease can occur without the principles of Ayurveda (Vata, Pitta, Kapha), ensuring each of these areas can be influenced by diet alone, making all illnesses responsive through special treatment through the use of Ayurveda. This does not indicate that Ayurvedic medicine can cure everything. Some illnesses can only be managed.

There is some evidence that the English cut the fingers of "Ayurvedic Marma practitioners" and suppressed totally Ayurvedic practices and teachings during their rule beginning in the 17th century. Ayurveda involves the animal, mineral, and plant kingdoms. The strongest of Ayurvedic remedies are not allowed in the United States. It is true that Dr. Vassant Lad, a doctor of Ayurvedic medicine, known worldwide has written numerous books making Ayurveda more understandable for the Western world, correlated Ayurveda to Western medicine. Some believe he has somewhat altered or taught in a different manner from the original texts used in medical schools in India, even today.

HIPPOCRATES

Hippocrates practiced and taught medicine in the 4th century B.C., on Kos, a Greek island. He was seen as the father of medicine, in part due to the fact he paid such close attention to physical symptoms of patients rather than theory, but also because after he died, medical documents were gathered in Hippocrates' name. This Hippocratic Collection and Oath have become the cornerstone of allopathic medical science to this day.

Later, a Greek document, entitled, *On the Nature of Man*, which was thought to be by Polybus, introduced one theory that became standard throughout the European region, which lasted about 2 millennia. The theory said that humans consist of four humors. The substances are phlegm, black bile (or melancholia), blood, and yellow bile (or chole). Having more than required of any one is supposed to cause symptoms or traits. These are phlegmatic, sanguine, choleric, or melancholy characteristics.

In the beginning of the 3rd century BC, two surgical specialists working in the cities of Alexandria, Erasistratus, and Herophilus, made the very first work towards discovering the secrets of human anatomy.

CHINESE MEDICINE

A 1st century BC text from China, the Book of Medicine, or *Nei Ching*, talked about acupuncture. The underlying theory of traditional Chinese Medicine is the health cycle of energy. The cycle may be affected by blockages, and they might be considered as the cause or the symptom of sickness. Moreover, by inserting a very fine acupuncture needle into the energy path would better the energy flow by releasing a blockage or lessening the pressure.

GALEN'S MEDICAL KNOWLEDGE

The main doctor for the gladiators in Pergamum, in 158 AD, was Galen, a Greek doctor. Galen's knowledge of the musculature helped him to advise those who came to him to treat the outcomes of various operations. However, it was Galen's analysis of pigs and apes that he dissected that taught him how the body's organs were arranged. They become the foundation for Galen's reputation. Through his experiments, Galen overturned many set-in-stone beliefs, including the belief that arteries hold air. His mistake, which became the orthodox for medicine for hundreds of years, was that blood travels back and forth from the body's heart.

EARLY LATIN AMERICAN SURGERY

Surgery in Mexico - Different techniques were successfully used on various parts of the body by the Mexica ("Azteca") even before the Europeans. Arthrocentesis, the surgery to remove fluid from the knee joint was one of them. Mexica doctors performed this operation hundreds of years before it was tried by the Europeans.

BEGINNINGS OF ANESTHESIA

A manuscript holds the first description of an anesthetic, though similar drugs may have been used in the Alexandrian school of medicine 1,000 years earlier. The doctor was instructed to mix in a brass pot specific amounts of opium, hemlock, mandragora, ivy, and non-ripened mulberry. The mixture was boiled along with a sponge, until all the mixture was soaked up by the sponge. The sponge was then held to the patient's nostrils.

Early Dental Surgery

An Arab doctor, Abul Kasim, was the doctor to the Emir of Cordoba. He wrote *Al-Tasrif*, the first illustrated manual of surgery. It was widely used and copied during the Middle Ages. He is also the first surgeon to be interested in dentistry.

Locating Bodily Organs

Vesalius, a young medical student, went to lectures at the University of Paris. The lecturer explained Galen's theories of anatomy, while an assistant gestured to the corresponding examples within a cadaver. Sadly, all too often, an assistant was unable to locate the organ being mentioned. Vesalius decided to dissect corpses and trust in the evidence he found himself. Galen performed many of his experiments on apes. Vesalius displayed for comparison the skeletons of an ape and a human. He showed that often Galen's theories are true for the ape, but less so for man.

Vesalius decided to compose a new description of human anatomy, shown in new dissections and drawings. He had a method of ensuring accurate images in print: it is called the woodcut. His research kickstarted a new field of scientific study called anatomy. In Switzerland, Vesalius published a voluminous work, called *De humani corporis fabrica*, or *The Structure of the Human Body*. This work had great success, though it did anger the traditionalists who still subscribed to Galen's theories.

Early Military Surgery

Before anesthetics, surgery was limited. It was also disliked by doctors whose reputation was based on their connection to authorities rather than their clinical skills. The most popular use of the surgeon was blood-letting.

The inventions of artillery and muskets changed the type of wounds that were treated. Instead of clean cuts from swords or pikes, wounds involved torn flesh and shattered bones. Ambroise Paré rose from being a barber's apprentice to being the surgeon for the French kings. His most important finding was that the usual treatment of any gunshot wound (cauterization with boiling oil), did even more harm. Paré found more success when he dressed the wounds instead. Paré also used ligatures for sealing blood vessels to stop blood flow.

Amputation was the sole major surgery which surgeons at that time were able to perform. Incision into the abdomen or other cavities was, during that period, too dangerous to attempt. Samuel Pepys was "cut for the stone" in London in 1658. The operation took place in a large room. It needed to be a big room because the whole family had to be there in case the surgery was not successful. With no good pain-killer, the speed of the surgeon was the most important thing. Pepys survived the operation.

Discovering How the Heart Works

Then in 1628, a newly published book, by William Harvey, gave us one of the greatest breakthroughs in medical knowledge (related to the heart), perhaps until DNA. In this book, he illustrated a new theory. "Blood," he wrote, "does not merely drift." Until then it was thought that the blood contained in arteries and veins was different. The theory was that the arterial blood carried energy somehow connected with air through the body (close enough to reality for that period of time), and our veins brought food from the liver to our body (far less accurate).

Through dissecting dogs, pigs, slugs, and oysters, to name a few, and by logic, Harvey proved the body uses only one blood supply, and the heart was pumping. This cycle brought the blood up into the heart's right ventricle, sent it through our lungs into the heart's left ventricle, then back through our arteries to the different areas of our bodies.

Using Microscopes in Medicine

Marcello Malpighi, a professor at the University of Bologna, had been using microscopes in biology. One evening he shined the setting sun into his lens through a frog's lung. He saw the blood contained in tubes — he was the first scientist to observe capillaries. The missing link in the theory of circulation was found. Through the capillaries, blood from the arteries delivered oxygen to the cells and then went back to the heart.

Blood Transfusion

Jean Baptiste Denis, Louis XIV's royal doctor, conducted an experiment in 1667. Trying to save the life of a boy, weakened by blood-letting, he used a quill to insert into his veins about half a pint of lamb's blood. Later, in the same year, the Royal Society in London hired him for a transfusion of Arthur Coga, a student who was described as "frantic." Sheep's blood was inserted into his vein. The scientists hoped this might cool his own blood. A week later, Coga felt better. He received more blood, with no bad effects.

Jean Baptiste Denis successfully gave blood to several patients. But in 1668, a patient died. Denis was sued by the patient's widow. He lost the case, but was not found guilty of murder. The experiment fell into disrepute, afterward for the next three years, the public remained upset about it. In 1670, a law made transfusion illegal in France. No more was heard of the practice until it was attempted in 19th century England. But, it was still a dangerous operation until the human blood groups were identified.

Early Smallpox Treatment

Before the end of the 17th century, a dangerous procedure, possibly done already in parts of Asia, became frequent in Turkish medicine. The operation was inoculation to protect against smallpox. Inoculation is based on the observation that people who come into contact with an infectious disease and survive are thereby protected against it. Inoculation is a safety measure, but in the case of smallpox it is also a dangerous one. Matter from a lightly infected victim is rubbed into a scratch in the person's skin, to induce a mild version of the disease. Most survived the attack and were afterward protected.

Inoculation reached Europe because of Lady Mary Wortley Montagu, a young woman in London who contracted smallpox and survived. Later, she went with her husband to Istanbul. On the trip, she saw inoculation being practiced. She submitted her infant son to inoculation and he survived. Lady Mary had a second child, and she had her inoculated as well with equal success. Lady Mary began campaigning for this medicine.

18Th Century Medicine

The 18th century is known for advances in medicine based on observation. Some who recorded their work were professors; others were country doctors. Their work raised the scientific bar of medicine, creating techniques and medicines.

William Smellie, one of these early researchers, was the first obstetrician to scientifically study childbirth. Smellie gave midwives and students in London lectures on childbirth. He offered his help to poor women, provided his students might attend the birth. He worked out a scientific account of labor, including previously unseen details of the process.

In 1761, a book was printed in Vienna which offered the general doctor a useful new type of internal analysis. Leopold Auenbrugger, an Austrian physician in a military hospital had many patients with fluid in their chest. To find out how much, he used a technique from his childhood. Auenbrugger worked in a tavern as a child and was taught to judge the amount of wine in a barrel by tapping on the top. He found this worked on a human chest. Auenbrugger found the diagnostic technique called percussion. It was disregarded at first by medical professionals, but it became more used after the stethoscope was created.

Cowpox

In the following decade, Edward Jenner worked in a village and became aware of a local idea, that people who had caught a mild pox from cows' udders (cowpox), never caught the more dangerous smallpox. Cowpox is rare, and it was not until 1796 that Jenner got to test his theory. A girl developed cowpox symptoms. Jenner used her to inoculate a boy. The boy got cowpox and recovered.

Inoculation became even more established due to Lady Mary Wortley Montagu. Six weeks after the cowpox inoculation, Jenner gave James Phipps a conventional smallpox inoculation. Phipps showed no sign of being infected with smallpox. Variolae Vaccinae, which means "smallpox of cows," was Jenner's title for cowpox. The phrase leads to the word vaccination for this new form of inoculation. After a bit of opposition from the medical field, vaccination proved itself and its use greatly increased. In Britain, the annual smallpox death rate fell during the 19th century from 2,000 per million to less than 100. By 1980, after international programs, there was no evidence of smallpox around the world.

Early Stethoscope

René Laënnec, a physician in Paris, specialized in chest diseases. Two events in 1816 led to his contribution to medicine. While walking in a courtyard, he saw children playing with a strip of wood. A boy scratched one end; his friend, holding the other end to his ear, heard the scratch. Soon after that event, Laënnec had a female patient too large for her heartbeat to be easily heard but too young for him to press his ear to her chest politely.

Thinking of the boys, he rolled a paper into a tube. He placed one end on her bosom and held his ear to the other. Through the tube, he heard better than with his ear to the chest. He had created the stethoscope (from Greek stethos, or chest, and scopein, to observe). Laënnec constructed a wooden tube, about nine inches long with ends that fit against the chest and into the ear. He spent three years analyzing the weird sounds which reached him as he listened to patients breathe. Laënnec identified the sounds of different stages of bronchitis, tuberculosis, and pneumonia. His findings were published in 1819.

Listening to the body had always been with the ear held to the body. The stethoscope became the mediating tool. In 1852, the modern, rubber version was created, and from that point on a doctor was able to use both of his ears.

Cholera Investigated

During an epidemic of cholera, John Snow (1813-1858) was able to prove that cholera was transferred through water. Then, Louis Pasteur (1822-1895) was able to prove organisms caused disease. In the early 1800s, scientists thought that some living things grew spontaneously from nonliving matter. Between 1857 and 1863 Pasteur proved that theory was incorrect.

Pasteur also looked to cure chicken cholera. Pasteur instructed one of his co-workers to vaccinate chickens with the disease they had cultured. Through an error, the co-worker forgot to do it, and the disease was exposed to air for some time. Then, when he returned, the man injected the chickens, and they did not perish. The chickens were then vaccinated using a new culture and still lived. Pasteur realized the germs had been weakened by their prolonged exposure to the air. When the chickens received the weaker form of the disease, they became immune to the illness. Pasteur and his staff later used this discovery to vaccinate for anthrax.

Rabies

In 1882, Pasteur's team invented an inoculation for treatment of rabies. A team member dried the bones of several rabbits who had died from rabies. Pasteur tried giving vaccinations that were derived from spines to test the vaccine on animals. Later, in 1885, Pasteur had success when using the inoculation on a human boy. Pasteur later invented the method to sterilize liquids through a heating process (now known as pasteurization).

Other Vaccines

In 1879, Robert Koch discovered the organism that causes leprosy. Later, in 1882, he isolated the tuberculosis bacteria that transfers cholera to humans. In 1882, the diphtheria bacteria was discovered. Diphtheria immunization was created by 1890. In 1880, typhoid was discovered. A vaccine for the treatment of typhoid was later created in 1896. By 1884, the cause of tetanus and pneumonia also were discovered by Koch.

More Modern Anesthesia

Surgery was improved and eased by the discovery of anesthetics when Sir Humphrey Davy (1778-1829) discovered that by inhaling ether, pain could be relieved. James Simpson (1811-1870), from Edinburgh University started to utilize chloroform in the surgery theater around 1847. Later, in 1884, the use of cocaine for local anesthesia became popular. After 1905, novocaine was commonly used as a surgical anesthetic.

Joseph Lister, in 1865, developed antiseptic surgery, preventing infection by using carbolic acid on patients. German surgeons sterilized surgeons' clothes and hands and steam was used for sterilization of surgical instruments. Gloves, made of rubber began to be used for surgical purposes in 1890.

The Sphygmomanometer

The sphygmomanometer or blood pressure meter, monitor, cuff or gauge is still in use today to determine blood pressure readings. It uses a cuff that inflates which restricts the flow of blood, while a mercury or electronic or mechanical manometer measures the blood pressure. Used with a method to determine the pressure that blood is flowing. It means starting pressure, and ending pressure. Manual sphygmomanometers still are used today with a stethoscope to listen while watching a gauge.

The sphygmomanometer was invented by Samuel Siegfried and Karl Ritter von Basch in 1881. Later, Scipione Riva-Rocci invented one that was more easily utilized. Harvey Cushing invented a more modern version, in 1901, and it was quickly adapted for use within the medical field. Mass manufacture began in the US, by W.A.

Baum. The unit of measurement normally used to describe blood pressure is called millimeters of mercury (mmHg), which is directly measured using a manual sphygmomanometer. Normal blood pressure is considered 120/80.

Hypnotherapy Anesthesia in Surgery

In the late part of the 19th century to the early part of the 20th century, Dr. James Braid, a British board certified orthopedic surgeon, began the use of hypnotherapy to prepare his young patients for surgery. Far less scary than going into a hospital and facing an anesthesiologist in an operating room, using hypnosis helped the children eliminate their fears, and prepared them for their procedures.

After surgery, he furthered the hypnotherapy to improve their natural healing ability. He became known as the Father of Hypnotherapy. Although pursued by the Church of England for using "nonsense" in the medical field, he was strongly supported by other doctors. The statistics gathered, as a result of the surgeries he performed, in comparison to other surgeons of his time, showed tremendous benefits.

Modern Medical Advances

Medicine made much progress in the 1900s. The first indirect transfusion of blood was completed in 1914. Insulin was in use by 1922. The Electroencephalograph was first used in 1929.

The First Antibiotics

In the meantime, new medicines were being discovered, developed, and eventually used. By 1910 Salvarsan, the first drug was available to treat syphilis. Prontosil became available in 1935 for the treatment of blood poisoning. In 1928, Penicillin was discovered by Alexander Fleming. Later, in 1944, Streptomycin was discovered and used for the treatment of tuberculosis.

The Iron Lung and More

In 1928, the Iron Lung was invented. Then, Willem Kolf invented, in 1943, the first machine for use as an artificial kidney, a form of dialysis. The U.S. National Health Service was started in 1948. Then, Dr. Jonas Salk created the poliomyelitis vaccine. A vaccine for measles came about in 1963.

Modern Surgery

Surgery also experienced many leaps forward. The hardest surgeries involved operating on the heart and brain. Both were positively developed in the late 1900s. The first invention of an external pacemaker was in 1950 by John Hopps and, the first internal one was used in 1958. In 1968, the first successful heart transplant was performed and by 1982, the first artificial heart was in use. In 1987, the first heart and lung transplant occurred.

Laser Surgery

In 1960, the laser was invented and by 1964 was used for surgery of the eye. Fiber optics development, in the 1950s, gave way to endoscopes being developed one decade later. Infertility treatment methods also improved, leading to the first test tube baby being born in 1978.

Goodbye Smallpox – Hello AIDS

In 1980, the World Health Organization announced that smallpox was gone for good. However, a new disease, AIDS (acquired immune deficiency syndrome), was isolated in 1981 and took lives at rapid rate.

The Cat Scan & Magnetic Resonance Imaging

Computerized Axial Scanning or the CAT scan was introduced in 1975. Then, by 1983 the MRI (Magnetic Resonance Imaging) was in use.

More Discoveries and Inventions

By 1986, synthetic skin had been created and then by 1990, gene therapy was introduced to the public. To this day, medical science continues to make new discoveries.

CHAPTER TWO
The History of Pharmacology

Most of the users of herbal remedies indicate an anecdotal reason for success rather than any clinical evidence of their efficiency. But, botanical remedies are rooted throughout the world, in the process of healing and compounding, perhaps for thousands of years.

Ancient History

Otzi the Iceman, a 5,300-year-old mummified man, discovered in 1991, carried his own medicine kit with him, and it included items such as birch fungus, a natural antibiotic. His autopsy showed he had intestinal parasites, and so the birch may have been for his treatment of that.

We can only guess about the prehistoric caveman's use and knowledge of herbal remedies, but clues and logical research show that cavemen used plants to help them survive. These plants were greater than any food or medicine to the early humans, through their healing properties, plants may have been grown to connect humans to the spirit world.

From the beginning of written history there is evidence of the field of compounding. Compounding began and paralleled the history of man. Ancient humans learned instinctively, by watching how birds and animals took care of themselves. The use of cool water, herbs, leaves, dirt, and mud, a soothing poultice, were first applied to an injury or wound. By trial and error, early man learned what combinations of plants and mud best served him for a poultice. Later, he would use that wisdom to benefit others in need. Although the caveman had crude methods, today's medications, as you will learn, evolved from sources in the herbal world, sources that were easily within reach and used by ancient humans.

The Beginnings of Compounding

The ancient art and science of compounding medicines stemmed from the human desire to relieve pain and provide protection from injury and death. Man, learned about the uses of various organic and inorganic materials, and how ancient civilizations utilized the art of compounding substances meant for religious or spiritual ceremonies, hundreds and thousands of years ago. This included the making of scents (perfumes and incense, essentially aromatherapy), as compounds for staying healthy, improving health, treating illness, and in preparation of the deceased for the afterlife. Alchemy gave rise to a great fund of knowledge of medicinal compounding.

One Small Example

In the Middle Ages, a fungus called ergot poisoned people who ate bread made with grains overtaken by it. Ergotism was the name of the disease caused by ergot, and it caused convulsions and hallucinations. Later, ergot was used in Europe to stop postpartum bleeding and force abortions. Sansert (known as methysergide), a synthetic form of ergot, was a treatment for migraine headaches and various other types of recurrent and painfully throbbing headaches. Methysergide was once regarded as an effective treatment for the prevention of migraines, although it was not effective in the treatment of a migraine in progress. Sadly, it was widely abused during the 1970s. It was used in large quantities and put into hot tea. Users (during the hippie generation) would drink it to illicit LSD-type hallucinations.

Ancient Civilizations Begin Compounding

When humans started writing, they also began to document their knowledge of plants and compounding remedies. Thus, we have knowledge about the use of herbal treatments going back to approximately 3,000 BC. As different cultures developed, and trade routes were created, travelers observed and learned about the use of medicinal plants from other groups.

We now prepare and take some of the commonly used herbal medicines the same way our ancestors did.

Babylon

Babylon, the cradle of civilization, has the oldest known writings about compounding apothecary. Going back to about 2600 BC, there were priest-healers, also working as natural pharmacists and physicians, hand compounding minerals and herbs to produce medicines for health. Clay tablets have recorded disease symptoms, the necessary prescribed materials, and how they compounded for consumption, along with some prayer or invocation to the gods for good health.

Ancient China

The ancient Chinese pharmaceutical abilities seemed to come, according to legends, from Shen Nung (2000 BC), an emperor who searched and researched the use of several hundred herbs for their medicinal value. It is rumored that he tested many of these remedies on himself and wrote the original Pen T-Sao, a native herbal record of over 350 drugs. Shen Nung is revered, even today, by Chinese pharmacies as a patron god, who examined herbs, roots, barks of trees from swamps, fields, and forests. These herbs are still used in the Chinese process of herbal medicine today. Some of the herbal medicines included rhubarb, ginseng, podophyllum, cinnamon bark, stramonium, and ma huang, also known as Ephedra.

Humans have always been concerned about using medicinal plants. Often, they cause a bitter taste on the tongue. The tongue has been believed to be the detector of poisons. Medicinal plants have been widely known to cause harm as well as heal.

Star Anise is a popular Chinese spice, partially because of its licorice-like flavor that helps promote healthy digestion. Star Anise can be made into a traditional tea used to soothe colic. However, in 2003 the FDA announced a warning against the tea—because Chinese Star Anise was sometimes mixed with Japanese Star Anise, a poisonous species of the herbal remedy.

For over two thousand years, herbal treatments have been the main element of Chinese medicine. If you were to visit a Chinese herb doctor in China, you would find huge Jars filled with herbs that they would take handfuls and mix together for boiling to make teas to help ailing patients.

Ancient Egypt

The Egyptian pharmacy field and medical care traces back about 5,000 years. The most important record of the apothecary is "Ebers Papyrus" (from about 1500 BC). It is a vast record of approximately 800 prescriptions, which records approximately 700 recipes for drugs to treat various ailments. The ancient Egyptian apothecary was arranged by at least two levels including gatherers of herbs also known as harvesters, and the preparers of the medication who were called fabricating chiefs.

In reality, these were compounding pharmacists. In the setting of what was called the "House of Life," the "Ebers Papyrus" was most probably written by a scribe from dictation by a compounding pharmacist as he produced the compounded remedy.

THE MEDITERRANEAN

Ancient Greece

In about 300 BC, Theophrastus, one of the early Greek philosophers and a great natural pharmacist, observed the various medicinal qualities of herbs and minerals. He was labeled the "father of botany." His keen observations of herbal medicines were amazingly accurate, even based on today's knowledge of herbal therapies. He instructed students who walked with him in the wild, about observing Nature's remedies firsthand.

Northern Turkey in Ancient Time

At about 100 BC, the King of Pontus, Mithridates VI, despite his lifelong battle with Rome, made time to study intensely the art of herbal poisons, and how to prevent poisoning and how to counteract such poisons. It is rumored that not only did he use the poisons on himself, but he used prisoners as guinea pigs to test the theories of poisons and antidotes. He earned his fame through an herbal formula of antidotal powers, with Mithridatum, which maintained popularity for well over a millennium.

ANCIENT MEDITERRANEAN REGION – LEMNOS

The Use of Medicinal Clays

Clay, Terra Sigillata (Sealed Earth), was discovered on the

Mediterranean island of Lemnos before 500BC. Once, every year, this special clay was brought up from a hillside pit in Lemnos, overseen by government officials and religious dignitaries. They washed and refined it, then rolled it into a mass of the right thickness to be made into sheets. Then the government officials watched as priestesses pressed the official government seal into those sheets. After that, it was sundried. The tablets were sold commercially as a Trademark of Authenticity.

As shamans and holy men discovered, medicinal clays date back thousands of years. Moreover, the indigenous people of the world used, and still use today, clay for medicinal purposes. Clay is mostly used externally in health spas (mud therapy), and green clay (French style) is used in liquids to stave off parasites and bacterial infections of the stomach and intestines, as was also the clay kaolin (original Kaopectate), and bentonite. The first recorded use of medicinal clay has been tracked back to Mesopotamia.

ANCIENT ROME

Pedanius Dioscorides

As life evolved in the 1st century AD in Rome, there was a tracking and intensive study of the field of pharmacy by Pedanius Dioscorides. Pedanius traveled with Roman armies throughout the Roman Empire to study the flora that might be applicable for medicinal use. He made records of what he observed, and created a system of rules for herb gathering, storage, and therapeutic use. His *Dioscorides' De Materia Medica*, was the main book of reference material for herbal medicinal use in Europe from the 1st century until the 1600s.

Galen

Galen of Rome was one of those men whose names will be remembered forever in the field of pharmacological medicine. During the 2nd century, he practiced and taught Pharmacology and the science of medicine in Rome. His field was preparation and compounding of herbal remedies and was used by the Western world for almost 1500 years. His name is remembered for mechanical compounding, Galenicals. Galen originated the first formula for a cold cream for beauty as well. His procedures are still used in compounding laboratories today.

Roman Controlled - Syria

Pharmacy and Medicine are no better represented than by the selfless apothecary Damian, and physician Cosmas. They were twin brothers from an Arabian village, and dedicated Catholics, who offered both spiritual advice through religion and their medical wisdom to the ill (without any cost) who came to them. Their practice was in the seaport of Aegean, then a part of Syria, a Roman province. Their careers ended in 303, when they were crucified, stoned, shot by arrows, and then finally executed by beheading. Muslim dictator and Prefect of Cilicia, Lysias, ordered them put to death (along with their three younger brothers) for their unwavering faith. Many miracles have been attributed to Saints Damian and Cosmas.

The Middle Ages

The Middle Ages kept the remaining wisdom of Western apothecary and medicine hidden from the public, preserved behind high monastery walls from around 400 AD to sometime in the 12th century. Priests became scientists who were cloistered to learn flora and apothecary around the 7th century. The knowledge is documented in manuscripts from many of these cloisters and older records that were translated and copied for monastery libraries. Monks walked out in nature to gather herbs in the fields and forests, or simply grew them in their private herb gardens. After studying the library records, they prepared them for apothecary use to treat those who were infirmed. Today, some of these gardens still exist in monasteries from these olden times, in many European countries.

The ArabianInfluence

Early Muslims divided the field of medicine science from the apothecary arts with the pharmacist from the physician Thus opening, in Bagdad, at the end of the 8th century, privately owned apothecary shops. They kept much of the Greek and Roman knowledge of apothecary, from those they had conquered and martyred, and soon added to their compendium of knowledge the production of syrups, candies, distillation of water, liquids with an alcoholic base, and many ways of conserving their medications. The spread of Muslim culture throughout Europe brought the knowledge of blending herbs with mortar and pestle, otherwise known as the pharmacy.

The pharmacists often examined the goods of traveling merchants, including sandalwood logs, and they made available the sweets of sugar cane stalks for local children. While conquering, Muslims conquered Africa and Europe, they brought a model of their pharmacy which was adopted everywhere.

During the Arabian era of pharmacy, no study would be complete without mentioning the prodigy of his time, a Persian, Ibn Sina (980-1037) AD, who was known as Avicenna in the West. Great apothecary, physician, philosopher, poet, and diplomat, a true intellectual giant, he was favored by Persian rulers and princes. While secluded with a friend who was also an apothecary, he wrote his pharmaceutical wisdom that became known as the authority of Western pharmaceutical knowledge for over 700 years. These works are still influential in the East.

Middle Ages in Europe

The witches of the past must be credited with first using herbs for the treatment of diseases in the Middle Ages. They learned and understood herbs and their healing powers. However, when male physicians became the norm, they benefited from the Church's inquisitions and witch burnings. Male physicians then claimed the credit for this knowledge and over time, most of the herbs were ignored and no longer used.

Due to Arabian influences in Europe, pharmacies began to open around the 17th century. Earlier, about around 1240 AD, in Sicily and the south of Italy, pharmacy was distanced from the field of medicine due to earlier Arabian influence. Emperor Frederick II of Hohenstaufen, of Germany and King of Sicily, presented at his Palermo Palace, an edict to pharmacists to separate their work from those of the medical field, and provided them with regulations for their pharmaceutical practices.

The concept of an officially sanctioned Pharmacopoeia, which must be used by all the nations' apothecaries, started in Florence. The Nuovo Receptario, in the original Italian, became the legal standard throughout the country in 1498. It came from a major cooperation of Guild Apothecaries and the local Medical organization and was the earliest work of inter-professional cooperation up until that time. Those groups were privy to advice and guidance that was available from the Dominican monk, Savonarola, who was then, Florence's political leader.

To England – Middle Ages

In the Middle Ages, from Italy to England, the commercial trade of apothecary standard products, along with the spice trades, was big business. In England, the Guild of Grocers monopolized control over the Apothecary stores. Years later, Apothecaries allied with court physicians of King James the First, who were protected by "Beefeaters" wearing heavily padded clothing due to fear of being bludgeoned at any moment. Philosopher-politician-poet, Sir Francis Bacon, was granted a charter by the King in 1617 to form a separate organization. It was called the "Master, Wardens, and Society of the Art and Mystery of the Apothecaries of the City of London." The grocers were not happy about this. This was the first syndicate of pharmacists in the West.

Coming to North America - Canada

Louis Hébert, a young apothecary from Paris, traveled to the New World in the early 17th century, helping Champlain to construct the first settlement at Port Royal in Nova Scotia. Hébert handled the caring, well-being, and health for the early pioneers. While there, he raised native plants for use in drugs and managed the herb gardens. When trading, the Micmac Indians arrived. Hébert examined the herbs that they offered. Included in the Mimac's compendium were: Hydrastis (Golden Seal), Verbascum (Mullein), Arum, (Jack-in-the-Pulpit), and Eupatorium (Boneset).

Because the habitat was destroyed by British Red Coats in 1613, Hébert temporarily returned to Paris and his Apothecary work there. But, he returned once again to Canada in 1617, with his family. This time he was in Quebec, where his gardening ability earned him the name of Canada's first successful farmer.

The American Colonies – 17Th Century

The American Colonies held the hope of religious freedom for many of Europe's most wealthy families who were essentially not aligned with the conventional Church of England's religious practices. Massachusetts was their landing point. John Winthrop, from England, became the first Governor of what was then known as the Massachusetts Bay Colony. Because he could not convince British apothecaries and physicians to move to the Colonies, he studied and sought wisdom from British apothecaries and medical doctors in his letters. He, then, added a section to his small general store dedicated to these imported drugs as well as the ones harvested from New England plants. In 1640, at his house, he provided the "art and mystery" of the services of apothecary for his local constituents.

Marshall's Contribution

In 1729, an Irish immigrant, Christopher Marshall, opened an apothecary in Philadelphia. For nearly 100 years, this pioneer in the pharmaceutical industry was the leading retail store and producer of chemicals for use in the pharmacy. Its greatest use was as a supply depot during the Revolutionary War. Marshall's granddaughter, Elizabeth, was to become American's first woman pharmacist.

The First US Hospital

The first hospital in the Americas was in Pennsylvania and was established in 1752, 25 years before Independence from England. One year later, Benjamin Franklin gave assistance to both hospital and pharmacy development. John Morgan, the second pharmacist of the hospital, affected both pharmacy and medicine through changes that would be valued by developing pharmacies all over

North America. Primarily as a pharmacist, later as a medical doctor, he was an advocate for writing prescriptions and assuring the independence of both fields, medicine and pharmacology.

Meanwhile, Back in Europe

Chemist Carl Wilhelm Scheele was an important natural scientist with a deep interest in pharmacy and chemistry. Born in 1742 in Sweden, Scheele discovered many minerals and substances that have contributed to a better world. This amazing genius discovered chlorine, tartaric acid, oxygen, prussic acid, glycerin, tungsten, nitroglycerin, and molybdenum, plus numerous organic compounds we all use in life today.

Friedrich Wilhelm Sertürner gave us knowledge of the chief narcotic principle of opium, morphine, and the recognition of a new organic classification: alkaloids. Recognition followed him, and he relocated to a pharmacy in Hameln (Hamelin), Germany and continued chemical research throughout his life.

From Sertürner's experiments with alkaloids, in 1817, Pierre Joseph Pelletier, along with Joseph Biename Caventou, a French pharmacist, created emetine from ipecacuanha, strychnine and brucine using nux vomica, then later extracting treatments from Peruvian barks for malaria, (i.e., the displacement of cinchonine cinchona and quinine tree barks). They isolated salts in their purest form, clinically tested them and created production facilities. Many other findings came from their laboratory and pharmacy as well.

The roots of today's pharmaceutical industry are tied strongly to the apothecaries that blended plants; their history dates back to Europe's Middle Ages. The pharmaceutical industry, as it is known today, really originated in the 19th century.

Germany's Merck Pharmaceuticals was most probably the earliest company to move in the direction of today's industry. The company, originally a storefront pharmacy, was founded in 1668. In 1827, Merck began focusing more on scientific and industrial concerns, through the production and sales of alkaloids.

Switzerland later developed a similar industry. Before, a main proponent of the textile trade, Swiss manufacturers realized their dyes had various properties including as antiseptics and started to sell them in the pharmaceutical market. Before World War I, the unregulated trade of medicines allowed a less strict separation of pharmaceutical and chemical businesses than today. The companies sold patent products such as cod liver oil, toothpaste, and hair gel products, as well as medicinal remedies.

About the Same Time in the United States

Pennsylvania's pharmacists had two major menaces facing them. First, it was the decline of the pharmaceutical practice, and second, being discriminated against by the medical teaching staff of the University of Pennsylvania. Two meetings took place in 1821, where the pharmacists voted to form an alliance, which led to The Philadelphia College of Pharmacy. Sixty-eight pharmacists put their signature on the First Constitution, and the College opened on November 9th of that year.

The premier U.S. industry in producing medicinal cures through herbal remedies was from the Shakers, a religious group that was an offshoot of the Quakers. Started 1830, their industry peaked in the mid-1860s and fell at the end of the 1800s. The Shakers grew and collected about 200 varieties of plants. They dried, cut, and made them into "bricks," which they then wrapped, labeled, and sold to pharmacies and doctors around the world. The Shaker label represented quality and consistency for more than 100 years.

Around the mid-1800s, a need for better communication among pharmaceutical practitioners to create a stand for education, and to control the quality of drugs, led to the formation of The American Pharmaceutical Association. The Association still serves the pharmaceutical industry today. The Second International Congress of Pharmacy, which took place in Paris, France, in 1867, saw a great division of opinion regarding the creation of limitations on pharmacies.

William Procter Jr., who was the leader of the American Pharmaceutical Association, stated that "Public opinion is in America, a forceful agent of reform." Furthermore, he said, "there is not the slightest obstacle toward a multiplication of drug stores, save that a lack of success." Those statements led the forefront for the American path of pharmacy.

Procter had graduated, in 1837, from The Philadelphia College of Pharmacy. Moreover, he owned and managed a retail pharmacy and was a professor at the College. He edited the American Journal of Pharmacy for 22 years. After retiring in 1869, he continued as the editor of the Journal, residing next door to the College. In 1872, he returned to be chairman of the College.

In 1868, Dr. Albert B. Prescott taught Pharmacy in Michigan. However, he was criticized for abandoning the required apprenticeship process before graduation. In 1871, the American Pharmaceutical Association denied him credentials. Yet, his course and the University's pharmaceutical program were the pioneers of education. They defined major changes including laboratory, curriculum (which included a basic science program) and a rule that students become involved in full-time studies. Prescott's methods, which were once ostracized, were eventually adopted by most pharmaceutical faculties.

In 1820, the first "United States Pharmacopoeia" was created by the medical profession. As the first book of pharmaceutical standards by a respected source, it received immediate acceptance. However, by 1877, the "U.S.P." nearly dissolved because the medical profession had no interest in what they deemed as competition for their dollars. Manufacturing pharmacist and physician, Dr. Edward Squibb, went to The American Pharmaceutical Association convention and as a result, pharmacists created the "Committee on Revision" chaired by the noted hospital pharmacist Charles Rice. He was assisted by Joseph Remington, a pharmacist and educator along with Dr. Squibb. The "U.S. Pharmacopoeia" emerged with even greater importance.

Meanwhile, Pfizer founded in 1849, was first in the business of various chemicals aimed at healthcare. They grew greatly during the Civil War as the need for antiseptics and pain medications multiplied.

The Awareness of a Problem

Seldom did preparations of herbal pharmaceuticals (when made a second, third, or 100th time) have the same potency, despite the identical processing by skilled 19th century pharmacists with outstanding integrity. This was because the plants themselves varied widely concerning the content of alkaloid and glucosidal content. The response to the problem came from Parke Davis, a pharmaceutical firm, that standardized in 1879, "Liquor Ergotae Purificatus." Further methods of standardization and assaying content occurred, and by 1883, they released their list of twenty standardized products.

From 1855 to 1940, scientific researchers including Henry Rusby, led expeditions for new medicinal plants to South America. In 1884, on an expedition to Peru to acquire quantities of coca leaves, Rusby crossed the Andes, ventured down the Amazon River, and suffered many hardships. Luckily, he returned to the US with 45,000 specimens of flora. Included with those massive amounts of new drug plants, was cocillana bark, and other pharmaceutical discoveries, some of which are very important in medicine today. He eventually became the Dean of Columbia University's College of Pharmacy.

Western explorers learned from South Americans, who hunted with arrows dipped in curare. Curare kills by keeping the muscle tissue from having any contact with nerves, eventually causing respiratory failure. In 1942, two physicians modified its potency for use as a muscle relaxant. Then, the conquest of Central America brought the knowledge of the Central and South American herbal remedies. Nicholas Culpepers, the English Physician, shared the knowledge from the indigenous.

While some of these ancient peoples no longer exist, many of their plants and their uses for them do. Here are just a few medical herbs of the world and how they are used:

> Belladonna (Atropa belladonna), also called deadly nightshade, was once thought to have helped witches fly. It was used to soothe peptic ulcers and colic. Today, it is used in eye examinations to dilate pupils as well as affect the parasympathetic nervous system.

> Bloodroot (Sanguinaria canadensis) was used in Native America for rheumatism, fevers, and vomiting. Doctors using herbal medicines use it today for more or less, the same purposes.

> Cacao (Theobroma cacao), or chocolate as we know it today, originated in Mexico and Central America. Pulp made from its seeds was once used to stimulate the nervous system.

Coca (Erythroxylum coca) is known as the plant converted to cocaine. However, in folk medicine, it was used as a treatment to numb the effects of cold weather and for toothache pain.

Curare (Chondrodendron tomentosum) is native to the Amazonian rain forest. It gave hunters a poison they used to paralyze their prey. This poison comes from the alkaloid Tubocurarine, a form of which is currently used today during surgical operations to paralyze muscles.

Eucalyptus (Eucalyptus globulus) was used in the treatment of infections and fevers. Today, we know it contains eucalyptol, which helps to dilate the small airways of the lungs. This makes it often a key ingredient in Vicks Vapo-Rub and herbal balms for sore muscles and joints.

Foxglove (Digitalis spp.) is from Western Europe, where folk healers used it as a diuretic and for other purposes. Today, Foxglove is use in the production of digoxin and digitoxin, powerful medications for the heart. However, controversy remains over its use due to its toxicity in the wild.

Ginkgo (Ginkgo biloba) is used today in the United States because studies show it improves circulation to the brain and is also effective in dementia patients. The tree originates from China, where its seeds were used to relieve wheezing and to treat incontinence.

Ipecac (Cephaelis ipecacuanha), discovered in South America, was used for clearing problems in the respiratory system and stomach. European explorers used Ipecac in the treatment of dysentery, and this is its use today, along with treatment for bronchitis and whooping cough.

The papaya (Carica papaya) was used by Mayans in their herbal medicine. The papaya fruit, has the chemical papain, which is a protein-dissolving enzyme. It eases digestive problems and is sold as an enzyme in tablet form in health food stores worldwide.

Quinine (Cinchona) comes from the mountains in South America. Peruvians used it to treat infection and fever. Today, we realize that the bark of the Cinchona contains alkaloids that can remedy malaria.

Visnaga (Ammi visnaga) was used in Egypt to treat kidney stones and was written about in the Ebers Papyrus. Today it is still used to reduce the pain of kidney stones. It is also the key ingredient in an asthma drug.

Western yew (Taxus brevifolia) grows in the Cascade Range and was once used to treat rheumatism. In the 1960s, National Cancer Institute researchers were able to isolate Taxol from the yew's bark extract. Taxol ends the cell (including cancer cells) division process. The US FDA approved it as a drug in 1993.

Wild yam (Dioscorea villosa) originates in throughout the US and Latin America. History shows the Mayans and Aztecs utilized it as a drug for pain relief, and early US pioneers treated their rheumatism with it. Wild yam roots contain plant sterols, specifically Diosgenin, which, when synthesized, creates progesterone.

Yohimbe (Pausinystalia yohimbe) is found in western Africa. The bark was used to stimulate male sexuality as an aphrodisiac, and its use includes modern medicine for the same effect.

At the Same Time in Europe

In the mid-1800s an innovative genius in France, pharmacist Stanislas Limousin, introduced the medicine dropper, which is an accurate system of coloring poisons, and wafer cachets leading to the mass production of the gelatin capsule. The greatest of his inventions included a device for inhaling therapeutic doses of oxygen and the invention of sealable glass ampoules for the sterilization and storage of hypodermic solutions.

In 1894, Behring and Roux, discovered an effective diphtheria antitoxin. Scientists in the US and Europe rushed to produce it. It became available first, in 1895, saving thousands of children. Vaccinating horses with diphtheria toxin became step number one in producing the antitoxin. From then on, until 1955 with the release of the poliomyelitis vaccine, many biological products became available.

For 30 years, in the 1800s to the early 1900s, French pharmacologist Ernest Francois Auguste Fourneau was the director of laboratories at the Institut Pasteur in France. He specifically created arsenic and bismuth compounds for syphilis treatment. He discovered treatments for sleeping sickness and discovered lifesaving sulfonamide compounds. From his research also came chemicals with antihistaminic properties. His work led to several chemotherapeutic discoveries.

Antibiotics

Antibiotics probably were first discovered by Pasteur in 1877. However, from 1925-1950, the flowering growth of the antibiotic era – saw mass production of medications to fight disease. Fleming's great finding in 1929 of penicillin was severely underdeveloped, but later it was studied in 1940 by Florey and Chain. Due to the intense pressure to find a treatment for World War II infections, mass production began rapidly – and costs were reduced to 1/10 of 1% of the original formula's cost. From then on, extensive research continued to discover antibiotics to conquer human microbes.

A Strange, But Famous Story

Strange as it seems, the story of a pharmacologist, Dr. Emil Coue from France, included a high level of successes with his mixture of remedies, that he compounded from powders and herbs, mixed together in his pharmacy, with a mortar and pestle. He added mental treatment in the form of a mantra, which worked successfully with patients in his town of Nancy, France. So, successful was his practice, that one day, around 1918, the police came to his home, because there were thousands of people begging to be treated, accumulating on his front lawn and pouring out into the streets. Of course, the treatment of such large numbers of sick people was impossible.

He simply walked out to them on his front lawn and told them (and I am paraphrasing) to say these words, with their eyes closed, repeated hundreds of times a day – to themselves, silently, like a mantra. The words were: "Every day, in every way, I am getting better, better, and better."
The results were astounding. Patients from all over France came for his 'miraculous' treatments. Soon, it was noticed by doctors from other countries, especially Great Britain, who had come to learn the method.

The works of Dr. Coue are written in French and even British Medical history. He was invited to teach his method to the British Medical Association, where he was greeted with great regard and welcomed by the attending British physicians who appreciated this new and safer approach.

The British Medical Association loved the simplicity of his meditation/mantra, he was invited to the AMA – American Medical Association, where he lectured on pharmacology and the mantra that had, by that time, helped tens of thousands of people in Europe.

The staunch AMA stood in disbelief that the mind could have anything to do with disease, and he was laughed off-stage and virtually pushed to exit the U.S. as a fraud. Today Coue's work is known worldwide as an auto suggestive healing method that has had great success using a single mantra and is taught by self-hypnosis organizations including the world-famous Silva Method.

Then in the US – The Changes of Automation

During the time period, in between the two world wars, there were breakthroughs in the development of new pharmaceutical products. The first being insulin, which launched the new pharmaceutical industry as its first major product. The second came just around the time of World War II, and that was mass production of penicillin, a discovery that is perhaps unparalleled by any other pharmaceutical medicine ever discovered.

An international, government-supported, collaboration of industry and scientists, worked on creating the mass-production of penicillin for treatment of injured soldiers during World War II, which resulted in thousands of lives being saved. The manner in which penicillin was developed began a new way for the pharmaceutical industry to develop its medicines.

After World War II, socialized healthcare arrived in many countries including the National Health Service (NHS) in the UK, which enforced a more structured health care system. In 1957, the NHS created a non-competitive market, by fixing the price of medicines. This allowed a fair return on investment for pharmaceutical producers, which gave them an incentive to invest in the creation of new drugs.

In 1961, the Thalidomide scandal caused a drastic increase in the regulation and testing of medicines, and a change in the US FDA regulations. New laws implemented in 1964, required extensive testing and proof of the efficacy of drugs, along with disclosures of any of their secondary/side effects.

Henry Ford's automotive automation methods brought about mass production, and an increased amount of knowledge, to the new pharmaceutical industry. Research in biology and chemistry enabled potential drugs to be invented systematically instead of random discoveries and inventions. This "golden age" of development happened in the post-war boom.

A short list of pharmaceuticals developed during this time:

- The birth-control pill, introduced in 1960, was almost as impressive in the pharmaceutical industry as the release of penicillin, allowing sexual equality and the ability for women to control their fertility cycles and prevent pregnancy.

- Valium (diazepam), a benzodiazepine, was developed and then marketed by Roche in 1963.

- Monoamine oxidase inhibitor (MAOI) anti-depressants and antipsychotics followed shortly after that. These pharmaceutical products guided a new era of psychiatry, adding the effectiveness of biological treatments to the drugs used.

- The 1970s brought cancer medications, in the US government's "war on cancer."

- ACE inhibitors were released in 1975, improving cardiac health.

- Paracetamol and Ibuprofen were developed in 1956 and 1969.

- A shift began in the industry's focus, and in 1977, ulcer drug Tagamet became the first bestselling drug, earning its makers over $1 billion per year. Its inventors were awarded the Nobel Prize.

Although there were breakthroughs, many companies mimicked their competitors rather than facing the expense and risks involved in research, attempting to get market share rather than invent new pharmaceutical medications. For example:

> AstraZeneca's proton pump inhibitor Nexium (esomeprazole), which was released in 2001, is just a purified single isomeric version of an older drug which happened to be losing its patent at the time of Nexium's release.

Patents were problems for the new pharmaceutical market. The Hatch-Waxman Act in 1984 standardized generic production of pharmaceuticals in America, but some still-developing countries ignored existing medical patents anyway.

The industry's focus became marketing. Then entered the lobbyists and political action committees, who financially lined politicians' pockets to protect their commercial interests. Finally, they focused on attorneys to enforce patent claims on their property. Of course, these actions have made the pharmaceutical industry appear corrupt in the eyes of the public.

Companies have tried to waive high costs through outsourcing various processes, and later, through buying smaller pharmaceutical research companies.

However, those newer technologies, new pharmaceutical inventions, were really what promises a positive future for the drug producers themselves. The advent of computers in the pharmaceutical industry and biotechnology created great forward leaps in the development of new medicines.

The automation of the invention process and computerization of genomics caused breakthroughs to occur even faster. Beginning with insulin, genetic modifications have permitted the fabrication of human proteins through bacteria. Biological medications including the monoclonal antibodies suggest a new realm of increasingly targeted medicines that could affect humans similar to last century's phenomenal pharmaceutical discoveries.

Herbs Today

Today's herbs include yarrow, for colds, colic, and toothache; aloe, a laxative also used on wounds; cardamom for digestive tract infections, nausea and vomiting; and devil's root, which is used to treat chronic bronchitis.

Summary of Herbal Therapies

Over thousands of years, plants still retain their healing properties.

What was a healing plant or herb thousands of years ago is still a healing plant or herb, today. Because of their great confidence in their healing ability, witches and physicians of the old world had to know their herbs. Plants gave healing powers to those who studied them, used them in their practice, and respected their usage for the treatment of health problems.

Today, we can benefit from the herbal wisdom retained throughout the years. Looking back through history, we can enjoy those herbs that have retained their healing abilities through all time by learning about them ourselves.

Many of today's synthetic medicines owe their existence to herbs, plants, and trees, occurring in nature. Our first pain medication   is a derivative of White Willow Bark — aspirin. One reason the pharmaceutical industry synthesizes these drugs is due to a law that you cannot apply for a patent on anything that is produced by nature.

Thus, pharmaceutical companies create a similar chemically-structured product that duplicates nature's healing property of herbs, plants, and trees. They market it while hardly ever mentioning the herbal remedy and its benefits. Nature has been robbed of its due credit.

Currently the pharma industry is the richest industry in the United States and spends well over $5 billion annually on advertising and marketing alone. A great deal of this money goes into the seduction of doctors, providing perks for those who prescribe their brand of magic potions; many of these are relatively useless in treating problems, and never help with the root cause of disease. Often, these medications have serious side effects that sometimes result in death. For drug producers, they have a big upside to negative side effects, because they get to invent new and questionably better drugs to counteract those side effects that they caused in the first place.

Let's not throw rocks at modern pharma yet, as they have treated millions of people and reduced their symptomology of diseases for about 100 years, although the tide is turning.

The Recent Return to the Ancient Art of Compounding Medicines

Compounding of custom medicines had evolved over many centuries, but because of the mass production of pharmaceuticals from the 1950s forward by the massive pharmaceutical industry, stagnated for many years and compounding declined severely. Luckily, the science and art of compounding wasn't dissipated in time, although its use greatly diminished for the next half century. Instead, pharmacies became local drug dealers and neither a compounder nor apothecary.

The physicians of Functional Medicine today recognize the vast value of custom compounding medications for their individual patients, and now custom compounding pharmacies are cropping up in the medical community once again. The field of custom compounding requires considerable training, education, and expertise for the physician who compounds their custom medications for patients. It allows physicians to be able to return to a more please patient doctor relationship that emphasizes specialization of care through a doctor's apothecary abilities, or custom ordering medications from a custom compounding apothecary service.

Custom compounding of medicines is needed for a variety of reasons. A medication may not be available because of lack of demand, and the driving force of the pharmaceutical industry is profit, a great deal of profit. When custom medications are not available, the Functional Medicine practitioner must make them himself, or contact a custom compounding pharmacy to produce them for him. Custom compounding pharmacies produce variances in dosages from commercially available pharmaceuticals; still their work is more of producing medications that simply are not available at any pharmacies from commercial drug producers.

With the knowledge of secondary effects of commercially available medications, and the incidence of allergic reactions to gluten, fillers, artificial colors, that are used in commercial pharmaceutical products, custom compounding produces perfect products without chemical or side effects that can negatively impact a patient's health. Also, well trained and educated custom compounders can add flavors.

When a medication is made from scratch, it is actual far more pharmaceutically ideal for individual patient use. Because many patients have varying disabilities and some cannot even swallow large-size standard pharmaceutical medications, custom compounding can often make it available in small dose packets flavored to their taste from custom compounding pharmacies; or through more tolerable or preferred routes like skin creams, buccal troches, or suppositories.

The Demand for a 'Clean' Product

Compounded medicines are needed for a number of reasons. Pharmaceutical products may be unavailable on the commercial market, possibly due to a low demand because of low profitability for the drug. Alternatively, perhaps for lack of availability in the strength required. Moreover, while the pharmacists doing the compounding do alter dosages from commercially fabricated products, most of the products they make are not commercially available.

The point is, that through use of compounding, using herbs, and alternatives to pharmaceutical medications might be far better choices because we can understand nature's intended natural healing which flows more dynamically into the Functional Medicine protocols.

CHAPTER THREE
The Roots of Functional Medicine

*"If you listen carefully to the patient, they
will tell you the diagnosis."*

*"The good physician treats the disease; the great
physician treats the patient*

who has the disease."

- Sir William Osler
Functional Medicine Pioneer

Let's trace the beginnings of Function Medicine to its founding roots. You'll quickly realize it is not a new fad, and it is rooted in the most modern of medical science. Sir William Osler believed that a good doctor is one who listens to the patient, and will get the patient's diagnosis from listening and a doctor who treats the entire patient as a whole is a great doctor. He was one of the first professors of medicine to teach at the School of Medicine at Johns Hopkins University. Johns Hopkins is one of the U.S.'s greatest research and teaching hospitals.

The Functional Medicine model comes from the breakthrough work of seven innovators in the field of molecular medicine. These seven are known to be pioneers of this new restorative health paradigm. They are: Archibald E. Garrod, Gregor Mendel, Linus Pauling, Roger Williams, Abram Hoffer, Hans Selye, Bruce Ames.

These seven pioneers unknowingly cooperated in developing the parts and parcels of a system of understanding the whole human being, as one organism. Moreover, the synthesis of their work has improved our understanding of the human body, what factors influence our having optimum health, or the opposite, deterioration which leads to chronic, degenerative diseases and death.

HISTORY OF THE PIONEERS

Archibald E. Garrod (1857-1936)

- Medical doctor interested in biochemistry and genetics at St. Bartholomew's Hospital in London
- Key contribution: Genetics cause inherited diseases
- Publications/lectures:
  - 1908 – lecture: "Inborn errors of Metabolism"
  - 1909 – publication: "Inborn Errors of Metabolism"
  - 1931 – publication: "Inborn Factors in Disease"
- Studied:
  - Alkaptonuria (rare condition - urine darkens on exposure to air)
  - Not the result of a bacterial infection as originally thought
  - Frequently, in offspring of marriages between first- cousins (recessive inheritance - Gregor Mendel -see below)

Gregor Mendel (1822–1884)

- Moravian scientist and Friar
- Key contribution: Founder of Genetics.
- Studied: Cross-breeding of green peas for different traits. His concept of dominant, recessive genetic characteristics implied our characteristics are "locked in stone" at conception.
- Identified missing enzyme required for protein breakdown (metabolic enzyme)
- Coined the term "inborn errors of metabolism" to describe what he saw
- Ideas not recognized until the 1950s, when he was referred to as the "Father of Chemical Genetics."
- Quote: *"I believe that no two individuals are exactly alike chemically any more than structurally."*

Linus C. Pauling (1901–1994)

- Oregon State University & California Institute of Technology graduate
- National Research Fellow
- Key contributions: Electrons determine bonds between and within molecules; helical structure of DNA
- Publications/lectures:
  - Lecturer at California Institute of Technology
  - The Nature of the Chemical Bond
    - Electrons as the key player in bonds between atoms (both within and between molecules)
  - General Theory of Protein Structure
    - Proteins as coiled polypeptide chains
  - 1940 - A Theory of the Structure and Process

of Formation of Antibodies
- ◆ 1949 - Mechanism of sickle cell anemia
    - ▪ Genetic mutations can alter molecular environment and, therefore, physiological function in disease states
- ◆ For the lay reader: Vitamin C and the Common Cold, Cancer and Vitamin C: A Discussion of the Nature, Causes, Prevention, and Treatment of Cancer with Special Reference to the Value of Vitamin C, and How to Live Longer and Feel Better
- Studied:
    - ◆ X-ray diffraction to determine three-dimensional structure of crystals and other molecules
    - ◆ Electron diffraction via the study of quantum mechanics with Albert Einstein (electrons as 'bond makers')
    - ◆ 1930s – The interaction between hemoglobin and iron (protein structure)

- Key events:
    - ◆ 1925 – Graduated with Ph.D. advanced studies in chemistry, physics and mathematics from California Institute of Technology
    - ◆ Awarded Guggenheim Fellowship for 1.5 years study in Europe (Arnold Sommerfield Institute for Theoretical Physics in Munich; Niels Bohr Institute in Copenhagen; Zurich)
    - ◆ Awarded Presidential Medal for Merit for his work on an artificial substitute for blood serum
    - ◆ 1948 – Professor at Oxford
        - ▪ Discovered DNA molecule and helical structure (later proved by Watson & Crick)
    - ◆ 1949 - Established sickle-cell anemia was a molecular disease caused by a single amino acid

anomaly in polypeptide chains of the hemoglobin molecule
  - ♦ 1973 – Founded Linus Pauling Institute of Science and Medicine
    - Research into nutrition
    - Established orthomolecular science with Abram Hoffer
    - Worked on vitamin C and related compounds in combination with amino acids to prevent/reverse atherosclerosis and associated damage in heart attack, stroke, and peripheral vascular disease
- Only recipient of two, unshared Nobel prizes:
  - ♦ Chemistry
  - ♦ Peace (work on the population effect of neutron flux and carbon 14 produced by atmospheric atomic testing)

Roger Williams, PhD (1893–1988)

- Key Concepts: Biochemical individuality in terms of the molecular origin of disease
- Key studies:
  - ♦ Description of anatomical and physiological variations among people and how they related to their individual responses to the environment
  - ♦ Relationship between "biochemical individuality" and differing nutritional needs for the optimal function of different people (even identical twins).
- Human Genome Project (the 1980s) showed genetic structure was not rigid
  - ♦ Bishop and Waldholz ("Genome") / Simon and Schuster, New York, 1990:
    - *"Aberrant genes do not, in and of themselves,*

cause disease. By and large their impact on an individual's health is minimal until the person is plunged into a harmful environment. The list of common diseases which has its roots in this genetic soil is growing almost daily. How many human ills will be added to the list is unknown, although some contend that almost every disorder compromising a full and healthy four score and ten years of life can be traced in one way or another to this genetic variability."

- Dr. Williams pioneered the revolution in Biochemical Individuality
    - Genetic polymorphism: variation in function surrounding a specific genetic trait
    - Transformation of genotype to phenotype as a consequence of nutritional, lifestyle and environmental factors
- Recognized nutritional status can influence expression of genetic characteristics
- Publications:
    - 1976 - "Potentially useful criteria for judging nutritional adequacy" (with Donald R. Davis)
        - Observation on how nutritional status influences the functional expression of genes
        - Phenotypic characteristics (e.g. voluntary consumption of food, sleeping time after anesthesia, post-surgery weight gain, heating time after surgery, hair growth after clipping, voluntary sugar consumption, and recovery time after poisoning) influenced by nutritional influence on gene expression
- No such thing as a 'normal' biochemical profile – we are all unique
- Development of RDAs (Food and Nutrition Board of the National Research Council) assumes 'normal'

biochemical profile
- ◆ Questionable relevance to the concept of optimal nutrition based upon individual needs
- Dr. Williams' work paved the way for Rucker and Tinker (the University of California at Davis, Department of Nutrition)
  - ◆ Described the role of nutrition in gene expression and its relationship to biochemical individuality as *"a fertile field for the application of molecular biology."*
- Examples of nutritional status influencing disease patterns in relation to biochemical individuality
  - ◆ Ability the individual to detoxify both exogenous and endogenous substances
  - ◆ Control of blood cholesterol
  - ◆ Metabolism of the potentially harmful amino acid homocysteine
  - ◆ Response of certain cancer genes to diet and environment.
- Dr. Williams coined the term "genetotrophic disease"
  - ◆ Diseases resulting from genetically determined nutritional metabolic needs not being met by the individual, associated with disadvantageous gene expression
  - ◆ Variation in human biochemical function was far greater than nutrition and medicine recognized prior to his publications
- During a lecture, he responded to an inquiry as to why RDAs were insufficient for the definition of a person's nutritional needs with the simple insight: "Nutrition is for real people. Statistical humans are of little interest."
- Motulsky:
  - ◆ Many common degenerative diseases are the result of an imbalance between nutritional intake and genetically determined nutritional requirements for good health

- Simopoulos:
  - "Of all the recent scientific advances contributing to our understanding of the role of nutrition in disease prevention and the variability in human nutrient needs, the recognition of genetic variation as a contributing factor must rank the highest."

Dr. Abram Hoffer (1917–2009)

- Medical doctor
- Native of Saskatchewan
- Key Concepts:
  - Genetic basis of schizophrenia (with Ernst Mayer)
  - Effect of nutrition on schizophrenia
  - Co-discovery of Vitamin B_3 (niacin)
  - Development of first controlled clinical trials in psychiatry
- Key Events:
  - 2008 - Inaugural recipient of the Dr. Rogers Prize for Excellence in Complementary and Alternative Medicine (CAM) for his work using nutrition and vitamins to treat and prevent disease
  - Established Schizophrenics Anonymous (via close relationship with Alcoholics Anonymous Founder Bill W)
  - Worked with Linus Pauling on orthomolecular psychiatry

- Studied:
  - Challenged view of schizophrenia as a result of poor mothering
  - Developed treatment of acute schizophrenia through principles of respect, shelter, sound nutrition, appropriate medication and

administration of large doses of water-soluble
vitamins (i.e. vitamins B_3 and C)
How the body's overall health could be restored by
replenishing it with essential vitamins and minerals and
eliminating toxic foods

Hans Selye (1907-1982)

- Hungarian-born
- Key Concepts:
  - Study of biological stress as a "non-specific
    response of the body to any demand"
- Publications:
  - 1936 - General Adaptation Syndrome
    (G.A.S.) (published in Nature)
    - AKA stress syndrome
    - Three-stage syndrome:
    1. Alarm Reaction (preparation for 'Fight or Flight')
    2. Stress Resistance
    3. Exhaustion (following extended period of stress
       - aging "due to wear and tear)
- Studied:
  - Stress
    - Prolonged food deprivation to the injection of a
      foreign substance into the body, to a good
      muscular workout
    - Causal relationship with major illnesses such as
      heart disease and cancer
    - New ways to help the body efficiently deal with
      life's wear and tear

- In Selye's words, his discovery was just *"enough to
  prevent the concept from ever slipping through our*

fingers again; [making] *it amenable to precise scientific analysis."*

Bruce Ames (1928)

- Research group leader at Children's Hospital Oakland Research Institute in Oakland, CA
- Key Concepts:
  - Link between vitamin K and disease processes, including aging
- Publications:
  - October 2009 - Vitamin K, an example of triage theory: is micronutrient inadequacy linked to diseases of aging? (American Journal of Clinical Nutrition)
    - The body prioritizes the use of scarce micronutrients in favor of short-term survival at the expense of long-term health
    - Low Vitamin K intake is associated with heart disease, osteoporosis, and cancer as the small intake is prioritized to the liver
    - Patients taking warfarin/Coumadin (blood thinners) are not receiving sufficient vitamin K for optimal long-term health
- Key Events:
  - 2006 – First presentation of Triage Theory of Aging
  - February 2010 – interviewed by nutritional supplement trade publication, Nutra-Ingredients
- Dr. Ames:
  - "If you are short of iron, you take it out of the liver before you take it out of the heart because if you take it out of the heart, you are dead. But, the downside is, doing this causes long-term DNA

damage, which doesn't show up as cancer for 20 years."

- "If you are deficient for years your body weakens, DNA becomes damaged and you get sick and eventually die."
- "If you want maximum life span, your micronutrient needs must be met throughout life."
- "A triage perspective reinforces recommendations of some experts that much of the population, along with warfarin/Coumadin patients are not getting sufficient vitamin K for optimal function of vitamin K-dependent proteins that are important to maintain long-term health..."

- Current FDA recommendations for vitamin K (90 mcg/ day for adults) are based on levels of adequate blood coagulation, and fall short of optimal long-term requirements

With such great people and such dynamic research the history of Functional Medicine continues with modern-day doctors who have built the science and taken it mainstream.

MODERN DAY FUNCTIONAL MEDICINE EXPERTS

Here is a summary of the doctors who have dedicated their lives and careers to the advancement of helping others through Functional Medicine.

Jeffrey S. Bland, PhD, FACN, CNS

- Co-founded the Institute for Functional Medicine (1991)
- Fellow of American College of Nutrition (where he is a Certified Nutrition Specialist) and the Association for Clinical Biochemistry
- Served as Director of Nutritional Research at the Linus Pauling Institute of Science and Medicine in the early 1980s, working directly with two-time Nobel Laureate, Dr. Linus Pauling
- In 2012, founded the Personalized Lifestyle Medicine Institute (PLMI), a nonprofit organization based in Seattle, Washington, where he continues to serve as President
- President and CEO of KinDex Therapeutics, which researched molecules associated with genetic expression patterns in chronic diseases
- Has authored several books about nutritional medicine both for the healthcare professional and for the general public; he is also the principal author of over 120 peer-reviewed research papers on nutritional biochemistry and medicine
- Has self-published a monthly audio journal, Functional Medicine Update, for more than 30 years that is distributed to health practitioners in 36 countries
- Founder and Chief Executive Officer of HealthComm

International, a global company that became a leader in the development of medical foods
- Chief Science Officer of Metagenics, Inc.
- President of MetaProteomics

David Scott Jones, M.D.

- President and Director of Medical Education Institute for Functional Medicine, Gig Harbor, Washington
- Family medicine practitioner with emphasis in functional and integrative medicine 30+ years
- Recognized expert in Functional Medicine (nutrition/ lifestyle changes)
- Recipient of the 1997 Linus Pauling Award in Functional Medicine
- Past President of PrimeCare, (Physician Association of Southern Oregon - IPASO) Responsible for disease management projects - diabetes, congestive heart failure, asthma, low back management, depression, etc.
- Served as Chief of Staff at the Ashland Community Hospital
- Past President of the Southern Oregon Society of Preventive Medicine
- Editor-in-chief, *TEXTBOOK OF FUNCTIONAL MEDICINE*, published 2005
- Lead author of: *21st CENTURY MEDICINE: A New Model for Medical Education*
- Author: *Healthy Changes*, a 16-week Workbook, focused on health-risk reduction.
- Lectured at the 9th Annual Integrative Medicine Distinguished Lectureship: Personalized Medicine: Creating a Healing Partnership, in Portland, Oregon

- Chairman of Southern Oregon Society of Preventive Medicine, President since 1977

Dr. Sidney M. Baker

- Graduate of Yale University and Yale Medical School
- Board-certified in Obstetrics and Gynecology, Pediatrics, and Environmental Medicine
- In private practice in Weston, CT
- Co-author of *Child Behavior, Your Ten-to-Fourteen-Year-Old, Detoxification & Healing, The Circadian Prescription, Yeast Connection Success Stories: A Collection of Stories from People Who Are Winning the Battle Against Devastating Illness*, and *Folic Acid: The Vital Nutrient That Fights Birth Defects Cancer and Heart Disease*
- Peace Corps volunteer in the 1960s
- Former assistant professor of Medical Computer Sciences, Yale Medical School
- Former director of the Gesell Institute of Human Development
- Currently employed at Medigenesis, Inc. as Chief Medical Director and Chairman
- Practicing physician - biochemical and environmental aspects of chronic health problems of children and adults
- In May 1999, honored with the Functional Medicine Linus Pauling Award in recognition of Baker's pioneering work developing the underlying principles of functional medicine
- Received both his B.A. degree (1960) and his M.D. degree (1964) from Yale University
- Specialty training in Obstetrics and is Board certified in Pediatrics and Environmental Medicine

Leo Galland, MD

- Has received international recognition as a leader in the field of Nutritional Medicine for the past 20 years
- Board-certified internist and Fellow of the American College of Physicians and the American College of Nutrition
- Honorary Professor of the International College of Nutrition
- Author of more than 30 scientific articles and textbook chapters, including an invited chapter on Functional Foods in the Encyclopedia of Human Nutrition, 2nd ed. (Elsevier 2005)
- Has written two highly acclaimed popular books, *Superimmunity for Kids* (Dell 1989) and *Power Healing* (Random House 1997)
- Created the Drug-Nutrient Workshop
- Received his education at Harvard University, New York University School of Medicine, and the N.Y.U.-Bellevue Medical Center (internal medicine)
- Has held faculty positions at New York University, Rockefeller University, the Albert Einstein College of Medicine, the State University of New York at Stony Brook, and the University of Connecticut
- In 2000, received the Linus Pauling Award from the Institute of Functional Medicine for formulating key concepts underlying the discipline of Functional Medicine.

David Perlmutter, MD, FACN, BIHM

- Board certified neurologist and Fellow of the American College of Nutrition

- Received his M.D. degree from the University of Miami School of Medicine and was awarded the Leonard G. Rowntree Research Award for best research by a medical student
- Serves as an Associate Professor at the University of Miami School of Medicine
- A frequent lecturer at symposia sponsored by such medical institutions as Harvard University, the University of Arizona, Scripps Institute, New York University, and Columbia University
- Has contributed extensively to the world medical literature with publications appearing in The Journal of Neurosurgery, The Southern Medical Journal, Journal of Applied Nutrition, and Archives of Neurology and is the author of many books
- Recognized internationally as a leader in the field of nutritional influences in neurological disorders
- Dr. Perlmutter has been interviewed on many nationally syndicated radio and television programs
- Serves as medical advisor to the Dr. Oz Show
- In 2002, was the recipient of the Linus Pauling Award for his innovative approaches to neurological disorders and the Denham Harman Award for his pioneering work in free radical science and its application on clinical medicine
  In 2006, was the recipient of the National Nutritional Foods Association Clinician of the Year Award
  In 2010, was awarded the Humanitarian of the Year award from the American College of Nutrition.

William R. Davis, MD

- A preventive cardiologist whose unique approach to diet allows him to advocate reversal, not just prevention, of heart disease
- Handles exposing the incredible nutritional blunder of health agencies advocating a diet containing "healthy whole grains"
- Founder of the international online program for heart health, Track Your Plaque
- Advocates a lifestyle in which all foods made from wheat are removed
- Articulates this approach in his book, Wheat Belly: Lose the wheat, lose the weight and find your path back to health
- Practices preventive cardiology in Milwaukee, Wisconsin

Eric Braverman, MD

- Director of The Place for Achieving Total Health (PATH Medical), with locations in New York, NY, Penndel, PA (metro-Philadelphia), and a national network of affiliated medical professionals
- Recipient of the American Medical Association's Physician Recognition Award
- Maintains Directorship of The PATH Foundation, a nonprofit research organization established to collect and analyze information concerning the diagnosis, prevention, and treatment of all aspects of brain biochemical disorders, with specific focus on the impact of brain illness on overall health
- Has published over one hundred research papers and

has participated in collaborative efforts with internationally recognized researchers
- Has published several books for the health-conscious readership

Mark Hyman, MD

- A family physician, four-time New York Times bestselling author, and an internationally recognized leader in Functional Medicine
- Serves as Chairman of the Board for The Institute for Functional Medicine and was awarded its 2009 Linus Pauling Functional Medicine Award
- Founder and Medical Director of The UltraWellness Center in Lenox, MA
- Formerly served as co-Medical Director at Canyon Ranch Lenox, one of the world's leading health resorts
- On the Board of Directors of The Center for Mind-Body Medicine and a faculty member of its Food As Medicine training program
- On the Board of Advisors of Dr. Memhet Oz's HealthCorps
- A volunteer for Partners in Health, with whom he worked immediately after the Haiti earthquake
- Has testified before the White House Commission on Complementary and Alternative Medicine and has consulted with the Surgeon General on diabetes prevention
- Has testified before the Senate Working Group on Health Care Reform on Functional Medicine, and participated in the White House Forum on Prevention and Wellness (June, 2009)
- With Drs. Dean Ornish and Michael Roizen, crafted and helped to introduce the Take Back Your Health Act of

2009 into the United States Senate, to provide for reimbursement of lifestyle treatment of chronic disease
- He continues to work in Washington on health reform
- He was recently awarded The Council on Litigation Management's 2010 Professionalism Award
- Received the American College of Nutrition 2009 Communication and Media Award for his contribution to promoting better understanding of nutrition science
- Has been featured on 60 Minutes, Larry King Live, CNN, and MSNBC

Pamela W. Smith, MD, MPH

- Twenty years of practice as an emergency room physician at the Detroit Medical Center
- A diplomat of the Board of the American Academy of Anti- Aging Physicians and an internationally known speaker and author on the subject of Metabolic, Anti-Aging, and Functional Medicine
- Holds a Master's in Public Health degree along with a Master's Degree in Metabolic and Nutritional Science
- Has been featured on CNN, PBS, and other television channels
- Has been interviewed in numerous consumer magazines, and has hosted her own radio show
- Currently the Director of the Center for Healthy Living and Longevity and the founder and Director of The Fellowship in Metabolic, Anti-Aging, and Functional Medicine
- Director of the Master's Program in Metabolic and Nutritional Medicine at the University of South Florida School of Medicine
- Author of best-selling books

Edward Conley, MD

- One of the most experienced CFIDS/FMS and autoimmune physicians in the world
- In 1987, was a nationally recognized sports medicine physician having served as camp physician for the U.S. Olympic Training Camp at Lake Placid
- Founded the Fatigue, Fibromyalgia, and Autoimmune Clinic and has treated thousands of people from all over the States and the world
- Board-certified Assistant Clinical Professor of Medicine at Michigan State University
- Best-selling author and featured on two national Public TV specials: Secrets to Reducing Fatigue (1999) and Secrets to Reducing Your Breast Cancer Risk (2004)
- A pioneer in the integrative treatment of CFIDS/FMS and autoimmune diseases, which combines the best of traditional medicine with holistic therapy
- Has conducted ground-breaking research, such as the role of HHV-6 in CFIDS, and has appeared on over 500 radio and TV programs throughout the U.S

Stephen T. Sinatra, MD, FACC, FACN, CNS, CBT

- Board-certified cardiologist, certified bioenergetic psychotherapist, and certified nutrition and anti-aging specialist
- Has lectured and facilitated workshops worldwide and has authored several publications and medical periodicals
- Has been a featured guest on many national radio

and television shows

- Has become well-known for his integration of conventional medicine with complementary nutritional and psychological therapies that help heal the heart
- Fellow in the American College of Cardiology and the American College of Nutrition, and served two four-year terms as the Chief of Cardiology at Manchester Memorial Hospital, where he had previously been Director of Medical Education for 18 years
- Has formulated a line of nutraceuticals designed to help outline a preventative path to health and well-being for not only his patients, but for the general population
- Has written many books including *Lower Your Blood Pressure in Eight Weeks* (2003), *The Sinatra Solution: Metabolic Cardiology* (2005, 2008, 2011), and *Reverse Heart Disease Now* (2007). His latest books include *The Healing Kitchen* (2010), *Earthing: The Most Important Health Discovery Ever?* (2010), *The Great Cholesterol Myth* (2012), and *The Great Cholesterol Myth Cookbook* (2014)
- Began writing a national newsletter in 1995 entitled HeartSense, which later became Heart, Health & Nutrition
- Dr. Sinatra's corresponding commercial website, DrSinatra.com reaches a wide range of people and offers advice on a large array of topics on healing and health
- Is adjunct faculty at the University of Connecticut (Assistant Clinical Professor of Medicine) and a member of the Dean's Council at his alma mater, Albany Medical School

Sanford Levy, MD, FACP, ABIHM

- Internist in practice in Buffalo, New York. His office practice is a self-pay specialty practice of integrative and holistic medicine;
- Has achieved prestigious fellowship in the American College of Physicians;
- Is board certified in Internal Medicine (1989) and Integrative Holistic Medicine (2003)
- Served on the Board of Directors of the American Holistic Medical Association (AHMA) and the American Board of Integrative Holistic Medicine (ABIHM)
- Currently on the Board of Directors of the Academy of Integrative Health & Medicine (AIHM)
- Is a 1986 graduate of the University of Buffalo Medical School, a volunteer faculty at the school, and a clinical associate professor of medicine

Bethany Hays, MD, FACOG

- Is a practicing obstetrician-gynecologist with a career-long passion for finding the best forms of healing and to incorporate them into her practice.
- Ten years ago, that dream came to a new level of realization in the opening of True North, a center for health and healing in Falmouth, Maine. This unique integrative practice has been created by a group of practitioners of conventional and complementary modalities.

CHAPTER FOUR
The FM Wheel (Pillar) Key Support System

To improve health and create balance

Functional Medicine is a science-based protocol to become healthy – the natural way. It is 100% focused on the patient. Rather than testing for the cause of one symptom and treating patients' symptomatic complaints as isolated illnesses, Functional Medicine works through a process, often treating patients who may have a multitude of chronic symptoms, physiological system imbalances, and dysfunctions, in a unique but efficient way.

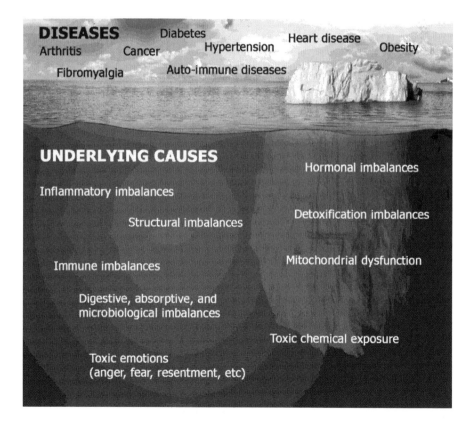

DISEASES   Diabetes
Arthritis   Cancer   Hypertension   Heart disease   Obesity
Fibromyalgia   Auto-immune diseases

UNDERLYING CAUSES
Hormonal imbalances
Inflammatory imbalances
Structural imbalances   Detoxification imbalances
Immune imbalances   Mitochondrial dysfunction
Digestive, absorptive, and microbiological imbalances
Toxic chemical exposure
Toxic emotions (anger, fear, resentment, etc)

As you might imagine from the iceberg graphic, you can see above the surface of the water only the symptoms indicating many of these common illnesses:

- Cancer
- Diabetes
- Hypertension
- Heart disease
- Autoimmune diseases
- Arthritis
- Fibromyalgia
- And, of course, obesity

That is like taking your child to a pediatric gastroenterologist and the child telling the physician, "I got an owie right here," pointing to the general area of the abdomen. That description of a symptom only gives the doctor a general description and no specifics from where to start helping. The doctor might start with a prescription medicine in liquid form, or send the child to the lab for a few tests, or to the hospital for major evaluations through a CAT scan (tomography) or something more.

How you feel, symptom-wise, is one thing; but, the symptom might be representative of several different problems interconnected, and might even be representative of several disassociated problems.

Moreover, receiving a prescription without testing does not always work to benefit you because below the surface, are the sources or root causes of the problem that are, all too often hidden and left untreated. You might liken this to putting a Band-Aid on a broken arm.

The reason this occurs is that the standard for most medical practices today treat only symptoms. And, office visits are but 10 minutes long after an hour or more of waiting to see the doctor.

Then, you get a prescription for medication or for a test, and return for another expensive office visit for follow-up.

The Benefits of Functional Medicine

In Functional Medicine, it goes without saying that one pillar impacts another. They all work together to create a balance, a homeostasis if all is well with you. The homeostasis is otherwise seen as a healthy and fully functional person. However, if something is out of balance, a system is not working correctly and disease and sickness is always the result.

Functional Medicine with its whole entity view, takes into consideration a patient's entire medical history from the womb and birth, to childhood and present health. It analyzes all the events of the patient's life including prior use of medications (antibiotics, anti- inflammatories, anti-hypertensives, steroids, etc.) and other drugs and/or alcohol use. Moreover, it takes into consideration prior life traumas (psychological, physical and emotional), your diet and lifestyle, and it continues from there.

Then, there is the analysis of the patient's nutritional intake, discovery of any vitamin and nutrient deficiencies that might be present, and the possible presence of environmental toxins in the patient's bodies. These are just some of the most important factors to be reviewed.

A doctor of Functional Medicine also looks at the patient's genetic hereditary factors from their parents. They view it not as a "booby" prize, but to see how those genes express according to the patient's choices in life. Perhaps you might view the genetic factors as a predetermined route that you must follow as if you ordered a TripTik® map from the AAA for traveling from point A to point B in your life. On the other hand, there is an emerging field of science called Epigenetics that looks more closely into this. The science of Epigenetics researches DNA sequencing traits on a cellular and physiological level. It explains how and why these changes in the cell's transcriptional potential impact us.

Transcription is defined as the transfer of genetic code data from one type of nucleic acid to another, with other factors involved. Unlike genetics that is solely focused on DNA sequence changes (the genotype), the gene expression changes our cellular phenotype of epigenetics due to other causes.

In Functional Medicine, we first analyze all the available history and other information from the patient's memory. Then, we look at all this data with this question in mind: How are all these symptoms or complaints expressing themselves as hints, or clues to what's really going on? Moreover, what are these clues trying to say to me, as your doctor, so I can help you?

It's my job, as your physician and a practitioner of Functional Medicine, to identify the cause of your symptoms that cause you to have health complaints. And, how can I work with you towards balancing the entire affected system so those symptoms complaints disappear naturally?

THE FUNCTIONAL MEDICINE TREE

Cardiology

Pulmonary

Urology

Endocrinology

Organ System
Diagnosis

Gastroenterology

Hepatology

Neurology

Immunology

Signs and
Symptoms

The Fundamental Organizing Systems and Core Clinical Imbalances

Assimilation
Digestion, Absorption, Microbiota/GI,
Respiration
Defense and Repair
Immune system, Inflammatory
processes, infection and microbiota

Energy
Energy regulation, Mitochondrial function
Biotransformation and **Elimination**
Toxicity, Detoxification
Communication
Endocrine, Neurotransmitters, Immune
messengers, Cognition

Transport
Cardiovascular, Lymphatic systems
Structural Integrity
From the subcellular membranes to
the musculoskeletal system

Antecedents, Triggers, and Mediators

Mental Emotional,
Spiritual Influences ◯ **Genetic Predisposition** ◯ Experiences,
Attitudes, Beliefs

Sleep & Relaxation

Enviromental
Pollutants

Exercise/
Movement

Micro-
organisms

Nutrition/
Hydration

Trauma

Stress/
Resilience

Relationships/Networks

Personalizing Lifestyle and Environmental Factor

Permission: Institute for Functional Medicine

FUNCTIONAL MEDICINE'S CORE PRINCIPLES

There are several core principles that guide Functional Medicine:

1. Having a total understanding of a patient's personal biochemistry, using both genetic concepts and the individuality of the patient's environment.
2. Get the necessary skills to understand any evidence supporting patient-centered treatment instead of the norm that is acute care — symptom/illness-centered focus to treating only the symptom at hand.
3. Research whatever is needed to have dynamic balance linking your internal and external: this includes body, mind and spirit.
4. Become familiar with and knowledgeable about all factors of inter-connectivity of core physiological factors.
5. Realize that healthfulness is a position sign of aliveness, rather than believing that it is simply the absence of disease in the body.
6. Accentuate all the factors that push you in the direction of developing a dynamically healthy physiology.
7. Support the patient's organ reserve to augment their being healthy and enjoying their longevity, not just their life span.

- Detoxification
- Vitamin Deficiencies
- Inflammation
- Intestinal Health
- Food Sensitivities
- Hormone Imbalances
- Stress Management
- Physical Activity

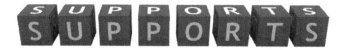

THE 8 FM SUPPORTS TO OPTIMUM HEALTH

There are 8 support concepts that we will discuss throughout this book, and we will be discussing each of them in great detail.

1. Vitamin and Minerals

I would love to believe that most people realize that vitamins and minerals are a must for our bodies to live healthy lives. Even though vitamins and minerals are important, our bodies are not designed to produce all the nutrients that are mandatory for optimal functioning of the human body. Instead, these nutrients must be obtained from the food we eat.

Unlike fats, carbohydrates, and proteins that are macronutrients, we know that vitamins and minerals are mandatory, and the body receives them in minute amounts. Because of that small quantity we need, they are called micronutrients. It is vital that your diet and food intake gives you the correct amount of micronutrients for your body's vitality. If you take in too much or too little, over time, it leads to disease.

Vitamins and minerals assist in human growth and physical development. Plus, micronutrients aid the body in producing energy from what we eat, building greater strength of your immune system, nervous system, reproductive system, etc. 26 micronutrients are needed in your body for you to maintain a healthful state of life. The body can produce 3 micronutrients by itself, the rest you must take in through food or supplementation:

1. Vitamin D is produced when your skin is exposed to sunshine.
2. Vitamin K is produced in the intestines by bacterial action.
3. Biotin is also produced by bacterial action in the intestines.

All other micronutrients required by your body must be supplied by your diet, and that often takes a great deal of understanding about what foods will help you gain them.

MICRONUTRIENTS

MICRONUTRIENT	DERIVED FROM	BENEFITS
Acetic acid	Vinegar	Slows digestion
Citric acid	Fruit juices and fruits	Inhibits kidney stone formation
Lactic acid	Probiotics	Assists the body's naturally occurring flora within the digestive tract.
Malic acid	Fruits and vegetables, especially apples	Beneficial for fibromyalgia and chronic fatigue syndrome; Can help with oral hygiene.
Choline	Eggs, brussel sprouts, broccoli, and shrimp	Important for normal brain health and development; Necessary to remove excess cholesterol and fats from the liver; Helps congenital heart defects in the fetus; Offers protection against inflammation.

Taurine	Meat, fish, and dairy products	Improves heart function.
Boron	Fruits like apples, oranges, red grapes, pears, plums, kiwis, sultanas, dates, as well as certain vegetables, avocado, soybeans and nuts are rich sources of boron. Chickpeas, borlotti beans, hazel nuts, currants, peanut butter, red kidney beans, tomato, lentils, olives, onion, potato wine, and beer.	Improves the natural ability of the human body to absorb calcium and magnesium.
Cobalt		Cobalt aids in the bodily process of using vitamin B_{12}, which is one of the foremost health benefits of cobalt; Has an effect on some of the vascular systems related to cardiologic function; May play a role in iron absorption.

Chromium	Brewer's yeast, coffee, tea, cereals, potatoes, peas, oysters, rye, thyme, processed meats, whole grains, and beer.	Helps metabolize carbohydrates; Monitors blood sugar levels; Helps stabilize blood sugar; Helps prevent hypertension or high blood pressure; Helpful in preventing memory loss and for treatment of Alzheimer's disease; Lowers the risk of cardiovascular disease; Increases heart rate while also helping ward off infections and protect cells from damage; Reduces hunger, which aids in weight loss.
Calcium	Yogurt, sardines, cheddar cheese, milk, orange juice with calcium, sesame seeds, tofu, spinach, and salmon (including bones).	Strengthens bones and teeth, aids in weight management and wards off PMS.
Copper		Helps maintain healthy white blood cell numbers and helps your immune cells better engulf pathogens.

Fluorine	Naturally found in water, Earth's crust, and various food products in the form of a negatively charged fluoride ion (F-).	Beneficial for teeth; Helps prevent bone loss; Provides strength to the enamel; Reduces acid production.
Iodine	Seafood, iodized table salt (sodium chloride)	Necessary for proper thyroid function.
Iron	Red meat, fish, and poultry; dark-green leafy vegetables, quinoa, legumes, eggs, and dried beans.	Helps make collagen, a connective tissue that joins body tissues together; Protects the body from infections; Required to make amino acids (proteins).
Magnesium		Helps build bones; Helps nerve function; Vital to energy production from food; Assists in maintaining normal muscle and nerve function; Keeps heart rhythm steady, supports a healthy immune system; Helps maintain strong bones, Aids in regulating blood sugar levels; Aids in normalizing blood pressure;

Magnesium *(Continued...)*		Assists in energy metabolism and protein synthesis; Linked to a reduction of conditions like heart disease, hypertension, and diabetes.
Manganese	Nuts, seeds, whole grains, legumes, and pineapples.	Important in the formation of bones, connective tissues; Important for blood-clotting factors and sex hormones; Involved in fat and carbohydrate metabolism, calcium absorption, and blood sugar regulation; Important for brain and nerve function; May be helpful in treating osteoporosis, arthritis, premenstrual syndrome, diabetes, and epilepsy.
Molybdenum	Legumes, including beans, peas and lentils, leafy vegetables, grains, nuts and liver; Mineral water or "hard" tap water may also contain molybdenum.	In animal studies, tetrathiomolybdate dramatically inhibits pulmonary and liver fibrosis, helps prevent liver damage from acetaminophen, and reduces heart damage from doxorubicin, a bacterial antibiotic; Tetrathiomolybdate demonstrates to be partially protective effect against diabetes.

Selenium	Found in a variety of foods, the richest sources being Brazil nuts, seafood, and organ meats.	Important for cognitive function, a healthy immune system, and fertility for both men and women; Works with vitamin E as an antioxidant in preventing free radical from forming and may reduce skin cancer risk and prevent sunburn.
Zinc	Oysters, toasted wheat germ, veal liver, roast beef, crab, pork loin, baked beans, lobster, beef patty, dark chocolate, lamb, peanuts.	Regulates immune function, diarrhea treatment, learning and memory, wound healing, and age-related macular degeneration.
Vitamin A	Fruits and vegetables.	Keeps skin and mucous membrane cells healthy and moist, which inhibits infection by bacteria and viruses.

Vitamin B1 (thiamin)	Organ meats (beef kidney or liver), egg yolks, spinach, kale, collard greens, corn, corn meal, fortified cereals, brown rice, wheat germ, nuts, and berries.	Helps regulate your appetite; Beneficial for your nervous and cardiovascular systems; Maintains health of mucous membranes through providing nutrients for cellular development; Delivers nutrients for improving health of nerve cells and neuron structure and function; Improves cardiovascular function through maintaining red blood cells and improving circulation.
Vitamin B2 (riboflavin)		Helps metabolize fats, proteins, carbohydrates, and amino acids.
Vitamin B3 (niacin)	Dairy products, fish, green vegetables, grains, and meat.	Reduces the level of harmful low-density cholesterol and increase level of beneficial high-density cholesterol; Can help avoid Alzheimer's disease, both type 1 and type 2 diabetes, atherosclerosis, osteoarthritis, hardened arteries, cataracts, and choleric diarrhea.

Vitamin B5 (pantothenic acid)	Cereals, meat, eggs, nuts, yeast, fish, and fresh vegetables.	Very important for metabolism, balancing hormones, and maintaining good health; Improves the health of the skin and nervous system; May be beneficial in treatment of some types of acne; Helps to metabolize carbohydrates, proteins, and fats; Helps make Essential steroids and one of the brain neurotransmitters.
Vitamin B6 (group)		Functions as a component of more bodily process than any other vitamin; Mandatory for producing and synthesizing many bodily chemicals. This includes enzymes, insulin, hemoglobin, histamine, dopamine, adrenaline, neurotransmitters, and prostaglandins. Helps to promote and maintain healthy immune function; Needed for brain and central nervous system function; Mandatory for maintaining nerve and muscle cell health;

Vitamin B6 (group) *(Continue...)*		Vital for the formation of both red and white blood cells. Helps to guard the heart by inhibiting cholesterol deposits; Needed for proper absorption of vitamin B12.
Vitamin B7 (biotin)	Biotin is found in certain cosmetic products such as shampoos, in multivitamins and sold as individual supplements.	Helps turn the food you eat into energy; Assists in having healthy eyes, hair, skin, and nails.
Vitamin B8 (ergadenylic acid)	Beans, nuts, whole grains, cantaloupe, and citrus fruits.	Helps liver process fat and keeps muscles and nerves working; Impacts the quantity of serotonin for the nerves in your brain; May help increase ovulation frequency and support weight loss, Influences cellular performance.
Vitamin B9 (folic acid)	Spinach and collard, turnip and mustard greens, asparagus, Brussels sprouts, tomatoes, and many types of legumes	Especially essential during pregnancy for the proper development of the fetus; Aids in prevention of congenital birth defects such as spinal bifida.

Vitamin B9 (folic acid) (Continued...)	including garbanzo beans, peas, lentils; and dried beans, including black beans, kidney and lima, grain products, rice, chicken and beef liver, citrus fruits, nuts, avocados, brewer's yeast, and milk.	
Vitamin B12 (cyan cobalamin)		Maintains healthy nerve cells; Produces red blood cells, DNA and RNA; Assists iron to function properly; Helps folate in producing amino acid SAMe, to control mood. Supports immune function.
Vitamin C	Citrus fruit, leafy vegetables.	Helps prevent colds and flu.
Vitamin D	Main food sources are animal products, fortified milk and cereals, and sunlight exposure.	Required for the proper absorption and utilization of calcium and phosphorus in the body, which are both essential to the health of the skeleton.

Vitamin E	Eggs, liver, nuts and seeds, some types of vegetable oil, and also in some fruits and vegetables	For cell growth and differentiation; For blood clotting; For immune function.
Vitamin K		Vital for proper blood clotting and healthy bones; Helps the liver store and convert glucose into glycogen; Beneficial to rheumatoid arthritis sufferers because it is thought to reduce inflammation of the synovial lining of the joints.
Carotenoids	Alpha-carotene is found in vegetables like green peas, broccoli, green beans, spinach, collards and turnip greens, as well as in pumpkins and other squash, carrots and sweet potatoes.	Beta-carotene is a precursor to Vitamin A; Inhibits the oxidation of other molecules; It protects the body from free radicals.

Types of Vitamins and Minerals

Vitamins come in two classifications. Water-soluble and fat soluble. These classifications are determined by the body's capacity to store them. Water-soluble vitamins include Biotin, Folate, Vitamin C, and the B-group of vitamins. All these are not retained in the body for any length of time, so they must be replenished quite often. On the other hand, fat-soluble vitamins are retained for months within the body's fat tissues and can be used as needed. Fat-soluble vitamins must be consumed on a daily basis, but the excess intake from using too many vitamin supplements may have a toxic impact because the body has a limited facility to excrete them. Be careful!

Minerals are also broken into two classifications. Trace minerals and major minerals. Major minerals are required by your body in greater quantity than trace minerals. However, you might need more than you think! Your body's need for nutrients will vary depending on many factors including:

- Your age
- Your level of sexual activity
- Other activity levels, body-building, sports, etc.
- Your current health status

When you are pregnant or ill – your nutrient requirements are higher. When this occurs, you can supplement your food intake to build your micronutrient levels through an increase of foods rich in micronutrients, by using fortified-foods, or using supplements. If you are planning to get pregnant, you'll need to boost your intake of Folate and Iodine, and most pre-natal vitamins cover that. If you are already pregnant or breast-feeding your infant, you'll need to supplement most of the vitamins and minerals you normally get, speak to your Obstetrician about that.

If you are a vegetarian, you'll need to increase your Vitamin B_{12}, Iron, Calcium, and Zinc. If you are an athlete, you'll need to increase Iron and your B vitamins. If you are in your golden years, if you don't have a lot of time in the sun, you'll need to supplement Vitamin D, and you'll also need to increase you Vitamin B_6, Vitamin E, and Zinc. Because that will help you build a stronger immune system. You'll also need Vitamin B_{12}, Folate, Calcium, and Iron because your absorption level will probably be somewhat reduced.

Factors that Affect Absorption

Your intake of food is not the only thing that determines your level of micronutrients. Absorption of the micronutrients by the body is vital so that they can be properly used. The absorption of these micronutrients is often affected by illness, pharmaceutical medications, drug or alcohol use, and interaction that might occur with other foods. If you have diarrhea, IBS (Irritable Bowel Syndrome), celiac disorder, or problems with your liver – it will impact absorption.

Medications and over the counter drugs including diuretics, steroids, laxatives, and antacids containing an aluminum compound also impacts the absorption of micronutrients. If you drink, coffee, tea, caffeinated drinks, you may be decreasing your ability to absorb Calcium, Iron, Copper, and Zinc, especially when you are drinking caffeinated drinks when eating meals. On the other hand, if you include eating other types of foods, especially citrus fruits in your diet, it will enhance absorption of Iron while you are eating citrus with Iron-rich foods.

Vitamins are vital for life. I have met people who say I get all the vitamins from my food. Moreover, when queried about what they eat, they often tell me they get an egg and sausage muffin for breakfast, a super-sized burger for lunch, and then eat pizza for dinner. I am not kidding! For some reason, people do not get that the human body is a mechanism, which requires regular maintenance, like our automobiles.

If you do not put in oil, transmission fluid, and gasoline – the car will not run. If you try to operate the motor without oil the motor will not work; if you do not have transmission fluid in it, it will not shift gears. Without the proper lubricants and fuels, they will burn up or freeze up and die. The same is true with human beings; we need our nutritious meals with the necessary micronutrients to live a healthy life.

If you look at only one illness caused by the lack of one vitamin alone, you might get the point. Vitamin B_{12} deficiency refers to a low blood level of vitamin B_{12}. Symptoms which could occur include:

1. Problems with thinking clearly.
2. Personality changes occur, i.e. depression, irritability, and even psychosis.
3. Abnormal bodily sensations: changes in reflex reactions, poor muscle function, and if you have existing pain, it could increase.
4. Inflammation of your tongue.
5. Declination of your ability to taste flavors.
6. Reduction of your red blood cell count.
7. Weakening of heart's functionality.
8. A decrease in fertility.

Without early treatment, some of these symptoms could become permanent with no possible resolution. Causes of deficiencies might be related to absorption problems of nutrients being processed and digested in the stomach or intestines; this causes decreased Vitamin B_{12} uptake, and the need to increase or supplement Vitamin B_{12}.

The absorption process may also be hampered by internal parasites, pernicious anemia, or chronic inflammation of the pancreas. Also, surgical removal of part of the stomach, side effects of some medications, or genetic disorders will affect absorption. Decreased uptake of vitamins might also occur in Vegans, or patients who have malnutrition. If a patient has HIV or AIDS, or a disease-causing breakdown of the red blood cells, a Vitamin B_{12} regime should be implemented as soon as possible.

The Effect of Cooking Foods

You can destroy vitamins in food by exposing them to heat, water, light, and air. If you want foods to remain nutritious and healthy, foods must undergo minimal storage time and processing. Methods used today to lengthen shelf life of fruits and vegetables often cause them to lose their nutritional value. Eating organic produce, fruits, and veggies, from your garden are the best. Be sure to store them properly, in a cool, dark place, until they are ripe and ready to eat. Eat them raw, steam them – and keep the nutritious value and delicious taste at maximum. Organic produce markets are popping up everywhere with delicious and healthy foods. Utilize them for the highest nutritional value.

When you cook foods in hot/boiling water, they lose their mineral value. To reduce mineral losses, utilize methods of cooking which use minimal water (e.g. steaming), better yet – eat them raw!

Foods vs. Supplements

Your body requires minute quantities of vitamins and minerals daily and normally these are furnished through your balanced diet.

However, some have greater risk of being micronutrient deficient. These include women who are breast-feeding or pregnant, chronic dieters or vegans, those with malabsorption issues or allergies, including the elderly, and also smokers, alcoholics, and drug users. People who have inadequate nutritional intake may enjoy the use of vitamin and mineral supplements; however, supplements should never replace a nutritious diet.

2. Inflammation

Out of the top 10 causes of death in the US and North American countries, seven of them are disorders caused by chronic inflammation including:

1. Heart Disease
2. Cancer
3. Chronic Obstructive Pulmonary Disorder
4. Stroke
5. Alzheimer's
6. Diabetes
7. Nephritis

Inflammation was once considered to be only an acute short-term reaction to injury of soft tissue which appeared only as a specific symptom, and almost always resolves itself fairly quickly, i.e. sprained ankle, strained back pain from overdoing sports, etc. However, that is not really the case at all. Today's scientists and physicians have discovered that chronic inflammation tends to be one of the greater issues in degenerative disease processes. There are many causes of inflammation.

It could be related to stress and dysfunction at the cellular level, or it could be related to excessive caloric intake; it might even be problems with elevated blood sugar levels. Recently chronic inflammation has been clearly demonstrated to have destructive capacity.

Low-level, chronic inflammation is extremely difficult to diagnosis and has a destructive side to it. Stress-caused inflammation, with our current acute care healthcare system, may go undiagnosed for years and years; it may advance to become the foremost cause of cellular death in the human body. Because of the fact inflammation contributes to the deterioration that is associated with aging, chronic inflammation in the elderly has been given a label ... inflammaging.

Without your ever realizing it, low-level chronic inflammation could be a danger to you right now without even knowing it. When working with a doctor who specializes in Functional Medicine, you'll learn about inexpensive blood tests that can determine the impact of any inflammation in your body. At the same time, you'll learn how to combat chronic inflammation and avoid the decline in health, that so many experience as a result of aging.

INFLAMMATION – A Process
Acute Inflammatory Response

Inflammation is the way our immune systems respond and adapt to tissue injury, infection, etc. Inflammation plays an important part in the metabolizing of many organisms. The most basic of acute inflammatory response can be activated through:
- Injured tissue (through various traumas, overexposure to chemicals or heat), or
- Infections: started by bacteria, parasites, fungi, and viruses.

There are four symptoms that represent acute inflammation: The first two - redness and heat will come from an increase in the flow of blood to the where the injury impacted your body. The third - swelling comes to the site of injury from fluid accumulation and retention. This is because blood flow increases in the body's attempt to heal itself. Fourth and last, PAIN. Swelling tends to irritate or compress your nerve endings near the site of the injury. This causes pain related to inflammation. Pain is often the most important symptom to make you aware of any damage to tissues. Additionally, any inflammation in a joint – gives another sign, functional impairment. This limits movement and forces you to rest and allow time to heal.

A controlled acute inflammatory episode protects you in several ways:

1. It prevents infections from spreading and damaging tissues close to the point of impact.
2. It helps the body to eliminate tissues that have been damaged as well as pathogens.
3. It helps the body repair itself.

However, one other type of stimulus is cellular stress. That leads to malfunction and causes chronic inflammation that doesn't benefit your health and leads to disease and deterioration (over time) via several different processes.

Cellular Structure Stress and Chronic, Low-Level Inflammation

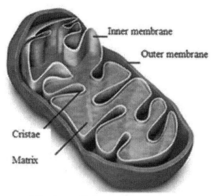

Mitochondria Inner Structure

This gets a little more complex here. Mitochondria (which are small cellular structures, also called organelles), which are found in the cytoplasm of eukaryotic cells (those are cells with a nucleus) have gained the nickname "powerhouse of the cell" because the Mitochondria produce ATP (Adenosine Triphosphate).

Diagram of Adenosine Triphosphate

ATP is a nucleoside triphosphate. A nucleotide triphosphate or NTP is a molecule containing a nucleotide (Nucleotides are organic molecules which are the monomers, or sub-units, of nucleic acids such as DNA and RNA) which are bound to three phosphates. Nucleotide derivatives are needed for us to live. They are considered the building blocks of nucleic acids, and have many other roles regarding cell metabolism, as well as, regulation and are used as a coenzyme by cells. It is sometimes referred to as the "molecular unit of currency" of transfer of intracellular energy. ATP moves chemical energy within the cells for the metabolism.

WHAT'S THE CAUSE OF Mitochondrial Dysfunction?

Mitochondrial Dysfunction is a risky problem. Moreover, it is caused by various environmental toxins, like tobacco smoke or second-hand smoke, increased stressors, and it is also a part of the normal process of aging in the elderly. One example: When mitochondrial energy is created, a byproduct of it is - free radical molecules. These damage cellular structures, triggering many genetic signals. This starts to create an inflammatory response. That inflammatory response as its end result kills cells. Moreover, it could be the opposite response; instead of killing cells, it sometimes causes uncontrolled cell growth that in most cases leads to cancer.

Aging - gracefully

When we age, it is due to a reduction of mitochondrial effectiveness and also an increase of free radicals (even though there are other theories of aging). Research indicates that the age-related abnormality of mitochondrial function causes chronic inflammation. (Dinarello 2011). With mitochondrial dysfunction taking place, inflammation is the result:

- Accumulation of free radicals causes the mitochondrial

membrane to become porous. Through the porous membrane, the molecules that would normally be in the Mitochondria seep into the intracellular fluid. That is where the cellular organelles are suspended. (the cytoplasm).

- There is a pattern recognition reception system in the Cytoplasm called PRRs. They act as a detection system and begin to create a response in the immune system against these intercellular pathogens, because they detect the leakage of mitochondria as a potential danger to the body. Once the system detects the threat, the PPRs produce inflammasome that activates another chemical (cytokine interleukin 1β) activating the immune system to destroy the damaged or infected cell.

This is a simplified description of how the mitochondria eventually causes cellular death. However, free radicals aren't the singular cause of cellular death from inflammation. Others include:

1. Circulating sugars, primarily glucose and fructose, are culprits as well.
2. Glycation is exacerbated by elevated blood sugar levels. (Witko-Sarsat et al. 1998; Vlassara et al. 2002).

Other biochemical inducers of chronic inflammatory responses are:

1. Crystals of uric acid can accumulate in joints during gouty arthritis. Elevated levels of uric acid are a risk factor for kidney disease, hypertension, and metabolic syndrome. (Martinon et al. 2006, Alvarez-Lario et al. 2011) Health Concerns

2. Oxidized lipoproteins (such as LDL), are a significant

contributor to atherosclerotic plaques. (Nguyen Khoa et al. 1999) Health Corners

3. Homocysteine (a non-protein-forming amino acid), is a marker and a risk factor for cardiovascular disease, and may be associated with increased risk of bone fracture. (Au-Yeung et al. 2006)

Together, these pro-inflammatory factors act together to create a perpetual state of chronic low-level inflammation called part inflammation (Medzhitov 2008). Chronic, low-level inflammation is the reason for many diseases, such as:

- Osteoporosis
- Cancer
- Type II Diabetes,
- Cardiovascular Diseases.

If you can target the numerous physiological issues that cause an inflammatory response, you could successfully reduce chronic inflammation, thus diminishing the impact of inflammatory diseases in your life.

Inflammation's Markers and Mediators

Here's a list of tell-tale symptoms of inflammation that have been used for medical diagnostics and research. Several are detectable through blood tests.

Tumor necrosis factor alpha (TNF-î) is a type of intercellular signaling protein known as cytokine, and is created by many kinds of immune cells responding to infection, damage or stress.

Excessive TNF-α may result in a chronic inflammatory disease. It is also associated with increases in blood clots (thrombosis) and a reduction in contractility of the heart. It may be responsible for starting tumors and their growth.

Interleukins are a family of cytokines that can be both pro-inflammatory and anti-inflammatory reactive protein (CRP) is an acute-phase protein and is one of several proteins that are rapidly produced by the liver during an inflammatory response. Elevation of CRP above normal base levels is not on its own diagnostic because it might be increased by several types of cancer. However, also other factors including gastrointestinal, cardiovascular and rheumatologic conditions, as well as infections. CRP elevation (which can be determined using a high-sensitivity CRP assay) is strongly linked with a high chance of Cardiovascular disease or stroke.

Nutrients Help Control Chronic Disease and Inflammation

First of all, inflammation is a healing reaction to something that happens to damage your body through trauma, etc. When inflammation grows to a point where it cannot be controlled, it is responsible for creating many different health issues. Inflammation causes discomfort and pain in some cases. However, good nutrition impacts the body in a healing way.

Many risk factors exist that might increase your potential of inflammation. They include:
- **Aging:** The older an adult becomes, towards their senior years, the higher their level of inflammatory molecules.
- **Obesity:** Fat produces those inflammatory molecules at higher levels that lead to a stronger inflammatory

response.

- **Diet:** If your diet is high in saturated fat then you'll have a higher level of pro-inflammatory markers. This is especially the case in diabetics or those who are severely overweight.
- **Low Testosterone or Estrogen:** Low sexual hormone levels repress production and secretion of man's pro-inflammatory markers.
- **Smoking:** Chronic smoking of any kind or any substance tends to increase the production of many types of pro-inflammatory cytokines. At the same time it reduces any production of molecules that are anti-inflammatory in nature.
- **Sleep Disorder:** The disturbance of your normal sleep process increases pro-inflammatory molecules during waking hours.
- **Glucose Levels being higher than normal** increase pro-inflammatory molecules as well.
- **Periodontal Disease** increases pro-inflammatory molecules also.

How Nutrients Help Chronic Disease and Inflammation

Bad nutrients have an opposite effect. If your diet is high in carbohydrate and/or low in protein, these will increase your pro-inflammatory response. This happens because refined sugar elevates your insulin level, and that increases the inflammatory process.

Allergens influence the inflammation process, especially with the common ones such as wheat/gluten and dairy – due to leaky gut syndrome and other issues of inflammatory disease. The diet in the U.S. and most Latin American countries involves a high content of animal fats, as well as hydrogenated and saturated fats. Add to that the level of sugar and carbohydrates and it impacts the inflammatory process. Adding to that highly processed foods and plastic bagged snacks with a high content of salt and preservatives, flavor enhancing additives and fillers, will further increase the inflammatory process.

This type of diet is low in fiber and plant-based food, which is needed for the proper operation of the digestive system. These foods have more Omega 6 than Omega 3 and tend to be high in wheat and dairy allergens. Those factors augment inflammation. However, a change to a proper, nutritious diet can reduce inflammation.

Enjoy Your Super-Foods

One of the challenges of modern times is to preserve the nutritional value of foods. This is mostly true for cultivated crops and foods. It is scientifically evident that the nutrient content of most of our food sources have declined over the last few years. Now more than ever we have to be conscious with our food choices since we might end up eating some things that are completely depleted on nutritious content.

Especially with the globalization of the food industry, fruits, vegetables, grains, and others are treated with chemicals to be able to preserve them to travel long distances, including to other continents, and over long periods of time. They have to endure hard climates and avoid decomposition.

Another sad and harmful issue is that whole-foods are consumed less and less. A large portion of people's plates nowadays (and specially snacks) consist of processed and packaged foods full of chemicals to preserve (or enhance) taste and shelf-life. For the most part people have lost the meaning of what a "real" food is like. "TV-dinners," those ready-to-microwave meals have very little real natural foods in them.

A group of foods that have maintained their nutritional value (for now) are wild-harvested "super-foods." These are natural products that for the most part are not cultivated by men but only collected from nature in an undisturbed environment. They are by definition organic, meaning without chemical fertilizers, pesticides, or the use of GMOs (Genetically Modified Organisms).

Another misconception is that any nutrient-rich food classifies as a "super-food." Some seeds and wild fruits are being promoted all over as "this is all you need to eat to survive." To be considered a super-food, and especially a whole food, not only does the food have to provide all or most of the micronutrients necessary for energy production and supporting life, but it also must have other "powers" like antioxidant products and enzymes, anti-inflammatory, detoxification, and others.

According to Barbara Swanson, an expert in Functional Nutrition, the three most complete whole foods are:

- Wild freshwater microalgae
Several species of edible microalgae exist in the wild or are cultivated. Some of the most nutritious ones are:

- AFA (Aphanizomenon Flos-aquae (Blue-Green)
- Spirulina
- Chlorella

- Tonic Mushrooms
All edible mushrooms used to be wild-harvested but over the last few years they have been also farmed. The most common used today are:

- Shitake

- Maitake
- Reishi
- Cordecyps
- Lions Mane

- Wild sea vegetables or seaweeds
- Dulse
- Wakame
- Ecklonia Kava
- Dunaliella Salina
- Nori

At the end of the book you will find resources to learn about these super-foods and where to obtain them.

Let's Talk About Avoiding Inflammation:

This is going to sound like I am lecturing you. However, it is vital that you listen to these concepts, perhaps more than once, so you can get on a dietary program that will reduce inflammation considerably.

1. If you have food allergies or sensitivities, and you know what they are – avoid them. If you do not know if you are allergic, get tested and find out what you are allergic to, so you can plan a healthy eating program.
2. Nature created plants for a reason. So, eat a whole food, plant- based diet that is high in fiber. This includes:
   a. Foods that are unprocessed and unrefined.
   b. Foods that are high in phytonutrients. These are anti- inflammatory plant chemicals.
   c. Consume minimal amounts of sugar or trans-fats.
3. Get your healthy fats from sources like nuts, olive oil (or olives), avocados, etc. Moreover, get your Omega 3 fats

from eating wild salmon, sardines, herring, microalgae, etc.

4. Exercise. We'll cover this in some detail in a later chapter.

5. Note the Vagus nerve. You must learn how to relax it. Because the Vagus nerve is the most powerful nerve in your body that helps relax the entire body and lowers your inflammation.

    Meditation is our recommended methods, and we'll cover that in a little while. Other methods to relax the Vagus nerve include deep breathing exercises or relaxing in a hot bath, listening to relaxing music.

6. You'll need probiotics, they are the good bacteria needed for healthy digestion in your stomach and intestines. There are many brands of bifidobacteria and lactobacillus species, be sure to locate a reputable brand with 10 billion CFU of bifidobacteria and lactobacillus.

7. Vitamins are mandatory. Most people do not live on a farm and pick their fruit and vegetables daily. By taking a multi-vitamin along with a mineral supplement, it will help you reduce any inflammation.

8. Use more of certain herbs and spices that have anti- inflammatory properties, like turmeric and ginger.

When you approach inflammation with a comprehensive program, as I just spelled out, you will reduce your inflammation and balance your immune system. Moreover, your body will thank you due to reduced inflammation because you'll feel better fast. As I said earlier on, if you can reduce inflammation by following this protocol, you might not need gastroenterologists, neurologists, or cardiologists in your future.

The Functional Medicine protocol is simply a method that makes our human bio-mechanism operate optimally. If we develop a medical specialty in inflammology – many other specialties will not be required.

3. Intestinal Health

The role of the intestines in overall health is underrated. Conventional medicine looks at the intestines as a place for mere absorption of foods and elimination of waste, which might be affected by ulcers, polyps, or diverticulitis, and in some cases inflammation diseases like Crohn's or ulcerative colitis. More and more, in recent years, clinical observations (like the hundreds of patients myself and other FM doctors have helped) and research, is pointing to the intestines as the cause of many systemic diseases, from migraines to autoimmune to neurological diseases.

Leaky Gut Syndrome – The Health Destroyer

Leaky Gut Syndrome (also known as LGS) is one of the biggest problems we face today. It is a cause of disease and bodily dysfunction and is responsible for perhaps more than half of all chronic health issues. This has been confirmed by lab tests. In Leaky Gut Syndrome, the epithelium of the small intestine's villi gets irritated and inflamed allowing metabolic and microbial toxins that are resident in the digestive system to enter the bloodstream. This compromises the liver, lymphatic system, and what's worse the immune system including the entirety of the endocrine system. This causes a multitude of incurable diseases where the body attacks itself. It is labeled as an autoimmune disorder. Inflammation can cause these health issues, (listed alphabetically):

- Asthma,
- Chronic Sinusitis
- Eczema
- Food Allergies
- Fibromyalgia
- Fungal Disorders
- Inflammatory Joint Disorders
- Irritable Bowel Syndrome
- Migraine Headaches
- Rheumatoid Arthritis
- Urticaria (Hives)

I've only listed a few of the more common diseases that begin as a result of the LGS, but there are more. LGS also is known to be a causative in uterine and breast fibroid tumor growth and PMS. Often LGS causes chronic fatigue and immune deficiencies in babies. Leaky Gut Syndrome is at its highest level it has ever been right now in worldwide populations. Previously, the only way that toxic bowel material could reach the bloodstream was through being cut or speared during ancient warfare, or through bullets penetrating the intestines in modern warfare.

Penetration of the bowel, during war, virtually always lead to septicemia that might have been treatable had the proper emergency medicine been available. Mostly, it was not, and septicemia led toward an early death. Other than due to trauma, our bodies usually had a rather effective barrier in the small intestine, allowing nutrients to enter but keeping out material carrying toxic microbial waste. This filtered out metabolic and microbial toxins that were present in the intestines.

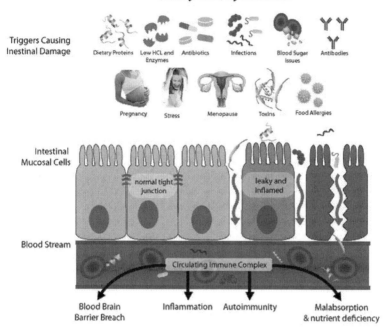

Now, it is a whole new ballgame, caused by the overuse of antibiotics and NSAIDs (non-steroidal anti-inflammatory devices). Mostly, it is the overuse of antibiotics, and secondly it is the use of NSAIDs.

Here's a list of some of the NSAIDs to be aware of:

- Aspirin (Anacin, Ascriptin, Bayer, Bufferin, Ecotrin, Excedrin)
- Choline and magnesium salicylates (CMT, Tricosal, Trilisate)
- Choline salicylate (Arthropan)
- Celecoxib (Celebrex)
- Diclofenac potassium (Cataflam)
- Diclofenac sodium (Voltaren, Voltaren XR)
- Diclofenac sodium with misoprostol (Arthrotec)
- Diflunisal (Dolobid)
- Doan's Pills, Magan, Mobidin, Mobogesic)
- Etodolac (Lodine, Lodine XL)
- Fenoprofen calcium (Nalfon)
- Flurbiprofen (Ansaid)
- Ibuprofen (Advil, Motrin, Motrin IB, Nuprin)
- Indomethacin (Indocin, Indocin SR)
- Ketoprofen (Actron, Orudis, Orudis KT, Oruvail)
- Magnesium salicylate (Arthritab, Bayer Select)
- Meclofenamate sodium (Meclomen)
- Mefenamic acid (Ponstel)
- Meloxicam (Mobic)
- Nabumetone (Relafen)
- Naproxen (Naprosyn, Naprelan*)
- Naproxen sodium (Aleve, Anaprox)
- Oxaprozin (Daypro)
- Piroxicam (Feldene)
- Rofecoxib (Vioxx)
- Salsalate (Amigesic, Anaflex 750, Disalcid, Marthritic)
- Mono-Gesic, Salflex, Salsitab)

- Sodium salicylate (various generics)
- Sulindac (Clinoril)
- Tolmetin sodium (Tolectin)
- Valdecoxib (Bextra)

NSAIDs actually cause inflammation of the intestinal lining allowing an opening of the space between cells and at times cause hemorrhaging.

There are other culprits that cause inflammation and LGS including drinking alcohol, inhaling formaldehyde (from new carpeting), side effects of chemotherapy, stress due to emotions ("I can't stomach that"), gluten/gliaden allergy, lactase deficiency, and abnormal gut flora (bacteria, parasites, yeast infections, etc.).

The First Antibiotic

As mentioned in Chapter Two, the first antibiotic discovered by Fleming was penicillin back in 1929. It did not get to be widely used until 1939, about the time of World War II, to save the lives of soldiers' who were shot or had surgery. Ever since the late 1950s, various forms of antibiotics have been prescribed by medical doctors for virtually every type of infection and inflammation, especially for treatment of children's ear infections, sore throats, bronchitis, etc.

Sadly, the majority of such infections are viral, and antibiotics do nothing to help the problems and instead, damage the intestinal flora in the body. Using them, in most cases in not necessary. In my experience, the use of antibiotics should be limited to hospitals or when the bacteria have entered the blood, bone, or organs of the body.

Effect of Antibiotics on Beneficial Bacteria

Antibiotics kill life forms inside the body, like bacteria. However, they are not intelligent and can cause damage. Antibiotics kill bad and good bacteria indiscriminately. There are almost over 2,500 different types of bacteria found in the small and large intestines of your body. Some of these bacteria are harmful, and some of them are extremely beneficial. Intestinal bacteria help the body in performing metabolic and some immune functions. The process of bodily metabolism is done by an enzyme secreted by beneficial bacteria. The process of metabolism consists of removal of microbial wastes and some hormones and toxins.

Functions of Bile

Bile is made and released by the liver and is stored in the gallbladder. It helps with digestion and assists your enzymes break down fats into fatty acids, which are brought into the body by your digestive tract. One of the functions of bile is to remove toxins from your liver. Bile enters the small intestine through a bile duct, after being store in the gallbladder. In your small intestine, beneficial bacteria break down the salt present in bile, and ensures the safe entry of this bile into the intestines.

However, when you take antibiotics the beneficial bacteria in the intestines are damaged or killed along with harmful bacteria. Due to the absence of these beneficial bacteria in your small intestine, bile containing harmful salts enters the large intestine. A hormone such as an estrogen metabolized by the liver is not broken down because beneficial bacteria in your small intestine are not present. If estrogen is not broken down, then it is reabsorbed into your body and can cause breast, uterine, or ovarian cancer.

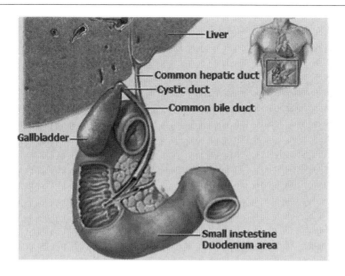

Effects of Antibiotics on Growth of Fungus:

Secondly, when you take antibiotics, it can promote the growth of certain bacteria, yeast and fungi. Most of the infections are due to a fungus called Candida Albicans. When the mucous membrane is damaged, then further protection is provided by a mucous secreted by the epithelial wall of the small intestine. If an excess amount of Candida Albicans is present, it results in Leaky Gut Syndrome.

Small intestine cells reduce in size due to secretion of Aldehyde secreted by Candida and thus, allows the entry of intestinal toxins into the blood stream. These toxins can damage organs including your brain.

Influence of Food Allergies

In a leaky gut, not only pathogens get entry, but also some nutrients from food. When your intestinal wall is not damaged, it allows only some digested and selective nutrients to enter.

However, when it is damaged, it allows toxins to come in with undigested food particles that enter the blood stream.

Due to this damage, your immune system cannot differentiate between the nutrients and toxins and marks them all as foreign particles. With that occurring, your immune system will initiate an inflammatory immune response in your intestinal wall. So, whenever a food containing these nutrients is eaten by you, it can initiate an immune response.

To avoid this inflammatory response stop eating foods like dairy products, eggs, gluten, and soy. Also, avoid these foods when the process of healing is taking place. You can eat meat, rice, garlic, and vegetables sometimes. It is important to differentiate what kind of allergy may be present. You can have an inflammatory histamine reaction due to either low stomach acid or caused by improper indigestion of food.

Involvement of the Liver and Lymphatic System

Usually, your liver works very hard in the metabolic process to remove metabolic waste from your body. Leaky Gut Syndrome allows the entry of metabolic wastes and microbial toxins into the blood stream. As a result, the liver works overtime cleaning the blood. With the passage of time, with those same conditions occurring, your liver may become sluggish and not detoxify these toxins any longer. Then again, these harmful toxins get into your bloodstream.

The human blood has its own mechanism to deal with these types of toxins. Whenever possible, your blood diffuses these toxins back into the intestinal fluids. However, this does not always occur. After, your lymphatic system will collect these toxins and transfer them to the liver, making the liver work even harder. If your liver is toxic, it will stop detoxifying these poisons. Ultimately these toxins begin to collect in your lymphatic system and cause chronic swelling of lymph nodes.

After some time, these toxins start to move into the connective tissues of muscles and joints furthest away from the lymph node, causing fibromyalgia. If they get entry into the normal cells, certain gene mutations can lead to the formation of cancerous cells in your body.

Immune and Endocrine System Responses to Stress:

Following are the three stages of stress to the immune system:

1. When you take antibiotics, they destroy beneficial bacteria present in the intestine. So, when some toxins and food antigens come in contact with the membrane of the intestine, the immune system becomes activated. It automatically releases an antibody called IgA antibody. This antibody will mark them as toxins living in your intestinal mucosa. So, ultimately white blood cells and macrophages detect these marked toxins for their removal.

2. As the liver and lymphatic system already have been invaded by toxins an immune system response is triggered.

3. As a result, your immunity will not work properly. This allows the growth of some virii, bacteria and fungi.

Due to a leaky gut your adrenal glands will not work properly either and will increase the secretion of cortisol. This cortisol secretion increase from adrenal gland initiates adrenal stress.

Involvement of the Digestive Tract

Sometimes, the condition of your small intestine is favorable for the survival of Candida. Attempts to remove them will fail if the status of your intestines remains the same. Lactobacillus is vital because it secretes lactic acid, which is very important to your body. When you take antibiotics, lactic acid is damaged and ultimately increases the alkalinity of your intestinal mucosa. Antibiotics taken for chronic illness decreases the productivity of acid in your stomach, and thus increases the alkalinity and the Candida survival rate also increases. In Leaky Gut Syndrome, patients often become malnourished and weak.

FIBER — A VITAL COMPONENT IN HAVING NORMAL BOWEL MOVEMENTS

Dietary fiber is not nutritious, but it is essential to our diets. The reason is, it goes through you, from your mouth to the anus, without absorption by the body. It provides an excellent vehicle to push excess intestinal waste out.

What is Fiber?

It is simply what's called "roughage," and it consists of edible plant parts that aren't really absorbed or digested by the body. It travels through the small intestine, and it continues to travel into your large intestine, to be passed out with our bowel movements. Types of fiber include cellulose, gums, pectins, non-polysaccharides, oligosaccharides (like inulin), and other associated plant materials including waxes and suberin.

Dietary fiber includes a category of resistant starch (in pulses, and seeds which have been partly milled seeds. It's call resistant because it's resistant to your digestive process in your small intestine and transfers completely unchanged into your large intestine.

In Summary

Inflammation of the small intestine stops the healthy digestion of what we eat and leads to poor absorption of the nutrients in our food. This also causes a cycle of abdominal pain, indigestion, and bloating, all which are symptoms of irritable bowel syndrome (IBS).

- If you were to absorb large, pre-digested pieces of food, it could result in food allergies and sensitivities, IBS, arthritis, fibromyalgia, and gallbladder disease.

- Inflammation of the intestines results in poor nutrient absorption, which leads to nutritional deficiency. When this happens, natural healing is impaired, and it can result in other symptoms, including abdominal spasms, angina attacks, sugar cravings, and even prostate inflammation or infection.

- When the detoxification system in the intestines is damaged, food allergies and chemical sensitivity, including sensitivity to medications, occur. This puts stress on the liver, making it difficult to handle required daily functions.

- When chemical additives and other man-made ingredients are eaten, the body struggles to process these ingredients, and new chemical compounds are produced in the intestines.

- There is a protective layer of mucus in the intestine, and inflammation damages it. When it is damaged, this increases your vulnerability to infection by viruses, bacteria, fungus, and yeast. Over time, these infections become resistant to treatment when the body's natural defense systems are weakened.

- All too often, this infectious process is mistakenly treated with more antibiotics. This just makes the situation worse because inflammation, and later further damage of the intestinal mucous lining, permits bacteria and yeast infections to go from the intestines into the bloodstream and spread infection throughout the body.

- When food antigens are activated by pre-digested nutrients that enter the bloodstream early, they attract antibodies. Those antibodies neutralize the value of the nutrient and in the process, damage the adjacent tissue.

Where Can You Find Dietary Fiber?

To give you a simple list, you'll find dietary fiber in fruit (oranges, grapefruit, lemons, limes, raspberries, strawberries, blackberries, pears, apples, etc.), and in vegetables (broccoli, green beans, garlic, peas, corn, onions, Brussels sprouts, artichokes, etc.), and in pulses (lentils, beans, chickpeas, etc.), and other places as well.

Different Types of Dietary Fiber

Dietary fiber is categorized by its content whether it is soluble or not. Both fiber types are in various percentages in substances that contain fiber. Great sources of soluble fiber are fruits, vegetables, and pulses. Other forms exist but aren't as healthy for the body because they are grain-based.

Dietary Fiber and Your Health

When you ingest dietary fiber, it moves to the large intestine. From there the fiber ferments, either completely or partially, caused by bacteria that is in intestines. This fermentation forms various by-products, including fatty acids and gasses. It's the actions of fermentation with those products formed which are so powerful in benefiting your health.

The major physiological effects caused by eating dietary fiber include:

- **Bowel function**
  Dietary fiber, especially the insoluble type, helps prevent constipation. It does this by increasing the weight of your stool and increasing the speed with which it travels through your intestines. The effect is improved when the fiber is also consumed with water. The short chain fatty acids, produced when fiber ferments through impact with intestinal bacteria, are a vital energy source for the colon, and may reduce growth and spread of intestinal tumors.

  Using dietary fiber to improve your bowel movements reduces your risk of disease, as well as disorders including diverticulitis and hemorrhoids, and it can also protect you from colon cancer.

- **Improving Your Blood Glucose Level**
  Eating soluble fiber slows down your digestion and the carbohydrate absorption, reducing the increase in your blood glucose after eating and improving your insulin response. That is beneficial for those with diabetes and helps them lower their blood glucose levels as well.

- **Lowering Your Blood Cholesterol**
  Studies have identified that dietary fiber is extremely beneficial in the prevention of heart problems (CHD – Coronary Heart Disease). Dietary fiber improves your blood lipid profiles. Isolated viscous fibers, including pectin, lowers the serum cholesterol and the low-density lipoprotein (LDL), as well as the cholesterol. Diets high in a mixed dietary fiber will protect you against coronary heart disease.

The benefits are clear: fiber prevents constipation (a natural detoxifying method), improves blood glucose level and blood lipid profiles and more. Eating fiber conveniently gives you the necessary dietary bulk without any additional calories, satisfying appetite and helping with controlling your weight. It is best to get all the benefits that fiber has to offer and to do that you should vary your sources of fiber. Fruits, vegetables, lentils and beans all provide you with fiber, as well as many other nutrients that are great for your health.

More good news: studies indicate that when you increase your fiber intake it reduces your risk of ever getting colorectal cancer. This is probably because of fiber's ability to increase material to your whole system of digestion, reducing the amount of time the waste takes to travel into the intestines and out the colon.

Human bodily waste often retains carcinogens, and so, it is in your best interest to get the waste removed ASAP. Increasing fiber decreases potential for intestines to be impacted by bacteria by removing it as quickly as possible. Additionally, if bacteria from the large intestine breaks down the fiber, as mentioned earlier, the by-product (butyrate) is manufactured which increases the change of tumor development in the colon and anus.

Newer findings indicate that fiber can also help protect women against breast cancer. Diets which are high in fiber are mostly low in fat, and that could explain the good effects of consuming fiber-rich beans, fruits, and vegetables since it's believed that fat increases the threat of cancer of the breast. Studies indicate that elevated fiber reduce or eliminate cancer of the breast through binding with the estrogen. Elevated levels of estrogen are potentially carcinogenic. Your liver is the organ that filters estrogen from the blood and sends them into the intestines where fiber pushes them out. Increased dietary fiber helps expedite the removal of potentially harmful excess estrogens. It is also indicated that fiber can protect you against mouth, throat, and esophageal cancers.

4. Food Sensitivities and FoodChoices

In general, there are certain groups of foods that should only be consumed, very rarely (or never if you can), and those are sugars and highly refined carbs, especially grains and most importantly wheat (white or whole grain). However, certain people have reactions to specific foods. They can cause many symptoms, at the beginning they might be subtle like bloating or headache but if the "insult" persists for many years they can affect systemic organs or part of the body and become diseases.

These reactions can be grouped into three types:

1- **Food Allergies.** These usually occur within minutes after eating the offending food and can manifest as a rash, swelling or breathing problems. They are immune-related and mediated by IgE (Immunoglobulin E). It is detected by history (for example swelling every time you eat shrimp), skin or blood tests. It is treated by food elimination, vaccines or anti-allergic medications.

2- **Food Sensitivities.** This is a less recognized type of reaction by the conventional doctors, but we see it all the time in FM practices. The reaction happens hours or days after ingestion, so the person does not see the causative effect and continues to eat the food for years. It can cause many symptoms, from locally bloating in the intestines, to migraines, joint pain, to inflammation that predisposes to Diabetes or Cancer.

It is mediated by IgG. It is detected by blood tests and the treatment consists of temporarily eliminating the food until those IgG antibodies disappear. This type of food allergy is probably more connected to Leaky Gut Syndrome than the others

3- **Food Intolerances.** These are usually related to the genetic lack of an enzyme to process a specific food. The most common is Lactose Intolerance where people do not tolerate dairy products due to a genetic deficiency of Lactase. There are four types, by the way, which you can see in the references provided at the end of the book.

Food Intolerance and Food Allergies

The majority of people enjoy variety in their diet without problems. However, a small percentage of them have issues with specific foods or ingredients that cause them adverse reactions, from simple rashes to anaphylactic reactions.

Food allergies or intolerances tend to cause adverse reactions. It is rumored that one out of three think they're allergic to various food ingredients. The truth is that food allergies affect only around one out of 50 adults. In infants and children, allergies are higher, somewhere between three and seven percent. Most every child outgrows their food allergies before they reach kindergarten.

Food Allergies vs. Food Intolerance

People can have adverse reactions to food, which they often mistake for a food allergy. Often, it is not an allergy at all. However, it in fact is caused by something else. Perhaps the food has microbial food poisoning, or perhaps it is a person having a psychological aversion to a specific food, or even a possible food intolerance to some ingredient that the food contains.

An allergy to a certain food involves a specific inability to tolerate a particular food or one of its components — and it causes reactions in the immune system. Allergens are a protein within the food that you might be reacting to, where a majority of those eating the food do not have a reaction. The allergen creates a chain reaction in your immune system that releases antibodies. Those antibodies cause your body to release chemicals, like histamines, which might give you a rash, a runny nose, choking, swelling, coughing, and other adverse reactions. Food allergies are often genetically acquired, and doctors and parents can usually detect them early in life.

One anecdote fits in here, a story of a young man who was, in his opinion, allergic to two things: eggs and salmon. A psychologist friend of his heard about this and told him he wanted to do an experiment. This took place in Salem, Oregon in 1990. The psychologist asked him to dinner, and before dinner, taught him some stress management exercises. He then continued to put the young man in a light meditative-hypnotic state in which he challenged the allergy.

> *"When you were young, you thought that you had an allergy to eggs and salmon and had reactions. Now that you are older, you have outgrown them. You've wondered what it would be like to eat eggs and salmon and not have a reaction. So, starting today you will no longer have any reaction to eating eggs and salmon and your desire to do so grows day by day and you will, from this day forth, begin to eat eggs and eat salmon comfortably with no reaction whatsoever. In a moment, you will open your eyes and will have a dinner of eggs and salmon."*

Simple therapy, really — the dinner of eggs and salmon went well with no reaction. Since they were friends for some time, the psychologist monitored the situation – and never again did the young man have a reaction. The only thing learned was that it was not a food allergy, but an immune system reaction, and that was easily overcome by the stress management and meditation-like hypnotic suggestion.

What Occurs When You Have an Allergic Reaction to Foods?

Our immune systems usually protect us from damage by foreign allergens and generate a response to eliminate them from the body. If you saw the movie "Hitch," there was a scene where Will Smith, playing the part of Alex Hitchens, had a response to shellfish when he ate Coquille St. Jacques. He starting choking, snorting, and had swelling of his face and ear. Quite funny in the movie, not funny in real life. That is an anaphylactic reaction.

An allergy means your immune system cannot handle what you ate, and an otherwise harmless food is determined as life-threatening. The body, manufactures antibodies, proteins that bind to other proteins, called antigens or allergens, to try to neutralize its effect and expel them from the body. This part is a little complex. The type of antibodies called immunoglobulin E (IgE) respond to the allergens and causes a reaction with mast (tissue) cells; also with basophils (a specific kind of blood cell). The mast cells reside just under the skin's surface, plus also in the linings (membranes) of our noses, respiratory system, eyes and intestines.

Histamines, or other elements including leukotrienes or prostaglandins, are then discharged from mast cells, causing allergic reactions. These adverse reactions usually come fast and furious, but are usually localized to one part of the body. Often, reactions take a few hours or even longer to appear after exposure. These are referred to as "delayed hypersensitivity reactions."

Luckily, most food ingredient allergies cause minimal reactions, but a tiny percentage cause harsh reactions that are often threatening to the allergic person. We mentioned anaphylactic reactions before, also called anaphylactic shock. Peanuts are famous for doing this in those who are allergic to them. The same goes for shellfish. If this happens, it is best to get to an urgent care or emergency room for treatment quickly. If anaphylactic shock occurs, the reactions are life-threatening, including a fast drop in blood pressure, and possible cardiac arrest, unless a physician administers adrenaline promptly to open respiratory pathways.

SYMPTOMS OF ALLERGIC REACTIONS TO FOODS

Respiratory	Asthma (difficulty breathing) Breathing difficulties Coughing Runny nose or nasal congestion Sneezing Wheezing
Skin	Eczema Itching (pruritus) Rashes or redness Swelling of the lips, mouth, tongue, face and/or throat (angioodema) Urticaria (hives)
Gastrointestinal	Abdominal cramps Bloating Colic Diarrhea Nausea Vomiting
Systemic	Anaphylactic shock (severe generalized shock)

Who Risks Having Food Allergy?

If a parent is allergic to a specific food, their infant could have double the likelihood of having the same food allergy. However, if both parents have the same allergy, the likelihood is four to six times greater. Breastfeeding for about six months usually reduces the risk of the food allergy, compared to infants who are fed formula.

How Prevalent is Getting Food Allergies?

Although one-in-three persons 'think' they have a food allergy, the actually numbers are far, far, lower. Studies have been done using double-blind, controlled food challenges where some participants have placebos. In these studies, it has been proven that only one to two percent of adults in our population have allergies.

Among children, it's higher. Most children outgrow their allergies by the time they are about three years old. When comparing long-lasting allergies to the ones that disappear with time, children's allergies to eggs, also to cow's milk end by age three. However, allergic reactions to fish, nuts, shellfish, and legumes usually last throughout adulthood.

The Most Common Food Allergy is ...

Cow's milk, while eggs, wheat (gluten), soy, shellfish, fruits, peanuts, and walnuts follow closely. Allergic reactions can come from virtually any food.

The Childhood Allergy to Cow's Milk

Infants and children are the most likely to have an allergy towards cow's milk, especially when there's a history of this allergy with one or both of the parents. The statistics show that anywhere from half a percent to four percent of infants born have a cow's milk allergy. However, the allergy usually decreases as they grow older.

Common symptoms of the cow's milk allergy include diarrhea and vomiting, but there are others that vary from one child to the next. Luckily cow's milk protein reactions are normally outgrown by the child at an early age. The prevalence in those over three years old and in adults is very low.

The allergen effect can be lessened by boiling the milk before drinking, or better yet, use evaporated milk — but never pasteurized milk. Yogurt, cheese, and other milk like buttermilk still have milk protein, so if you are allergic, avoid them. Once a milk protein allergy has been diagnosed, make sure your child has a healthy/balanced nutritional program, especially through the first few years of growth. Getting the proper dietary advice is mandatory so that the child gets their nutrient requirements including Vitamins A, D and B_2 and B_{12}, Calcium, and Magnesium.

Peanuts and Tree Nuts

Diagnosing and confirming a nut allergy is vital because it begins at an infant level, is a life-long problem, and can be fatal. Peanuts and tree nuts, such as pine nuts (pinons), almonds, Brazil nuts, hazelnuts, and walnuts can cause symptomatic reactions even if you do not consume them. Even skin contact or inhalation can cause a reaction. The reaction might be a rash, headache, or swelling of the tongue, but in its worst form, the reaction can be an anaphylactic shock. There is a potential for severe symptoms with any contact with nuts, and if allergic, the patient must carry injectable adrenaline (and know how to use it). Remember, nuts are used in recipes — cookies, cakes, gravy, stuffing, etc. in restaurants — and rarely is it posted on the menu. *Be careful!*

Other Food Allergens

Other foods commonly associated with allergic reactions include vegetables, fruits, sunflower seeds, poppy seeds, cottonseed, sesame seeds, mustard seed, soy products, eggs, lobster, crab, fish, and shrimp. Cooking and newer food processing methods tend to denature the proteins in these allergens, like high-pressure cooking, or enzymatic treatment.

Food Intolerance

Intolerance to certain foods may cause symptoms that are similar to a food allergy (including stomach cramps, nausea, and diarrhea). Food intolerance takes place when your body cannot properly digest a particular food. People who are allergic to food must eliminate the food from their diet while those who are intolerant to a certain food can often eat very small quantities without reaction. There are exceptions, such as people who are sensitive to glutens and foods made with sulfites.

The Most Common Food Intolerances are: Gluten and Lactose

Lactose Intolerance

Lactose, or the milk sugar, is normally digested by lactase while it resides in your small intestine. The Lactase is normally enough to digest lactose, breaking it down into simple sugars, for example, glucose and also galactose before it is then absorbed into your bloodstream. However, when your enzymatic activity is not functioning properly, lactose does not get digested, and it is carried forward to the large intestine, where it goes through a fermentation process due to the bacteria there. The responses are pain, gas, and diarrhea.

About 70% of the adults in the world have a lactase deficiency, although most of them descended from northern European countries where they do not have that problem. The amount of dairy consumed leading to intolerance symptoms varies. Some with low lactase activity in their intestines usually can drink a small glass of milk without problems.

Moreover, eating aged or hard cheeses, which have low lactose content, and products like yogurt can usually be eaten without much concern. That is probably why products like yogurt are so widely consumed worldwide, wherever lactase deficiency is a major problem. In fact, consuming small amounts of lactose-containing foods - such as yogurt with a meal usually can help improve tolerance in those who are sensitive to it.

Gluten Intolerance

As described earlier, some food intolerances do not entitle an immune response while others do. Gluten intolerance used to be considered a pure "intolerance" but in recent years research and clinical experience have shown that it is indeed an autoimmune disease. There are many degrees of gluten sensitivity, from mere bloating to more troublesome complaints like joint pain, mood changes to the severe cases of Celiac Disease (diarrhea, malabsorption, growth and mental delay).

I have a strict gluten-free policy for all of my autoimmune and weight loss patients. That combined with removing the foods from the diet that persons have developed IgG to, and replacing their missing vitamins and nutrients, you would be surprised to see how many patients I have helped (and maybe even cured) from autoimmune arthritis and skin diseases.

The well-known gluten intolerance occurs in intestines when your body cannot tolerate gluten. This substance is a protein created in wheat, barley, oats, and rye. The incidence of gluten intolerance, or celiac disease, is highly understated. Blood testing has shown that it is probably one percent of the population of European countries. Moreover, there are regional statistics showing that it is elsewhere as well.

Celiac disease, also called Celiac Sprue, is life-long. It can easily be diagnosed through testing. If someone with celiac disease eats food made with a gluten-based product in it, the small intestine's lining gets damaged and they have problems with digesting fats, carbohydrates, proteins, vitamins, and minerals.

Symptoms include:

- flatulence
- diarrhea
- weight loss
- weakness
- irritability
- abdominal cramps

In children, the problems with celiac disease can be very significant. Malnourishment is the number one issue because it leads to failure of the child to grow and develop. The only known treatment for celiac disease is a gluten-free diet, although there are others under investigation. Lists of gluten-free food products are included in the appendix of this book. When you remove gluten from the diet, the intestine begins to heal itself and results are seen fairly rapidly.

Although research is being conducted into identifying the specific cause and specifically which of gluten's amino acids might be responsible for celiac disease, it will be a while before this is known. In the meantime, quinoa is a good replacement for wheat.

Food Additives — Better Living Through Chemistry?

By law, all additives in food or food products must be labeled so that those with sensitivities can avoid them. For most people, they do not present a problem, although chemicals do not belong in the human body. Artificial flavors, colors, and sulfites are big problems for highly sensitive people.

Diagnosing a Food Allergy or Food Intolerance

Diagnosis of an intolerance or allergy to food can be done through scientific testing methods. If you think you might be having an allergic response to a particular food, speak to your doctor who can check if there is another possible cause. Then, testing can be accomplished, or referral to a nutritionist, or a physician who specializes in food allergies, if needed. Tests might include:

Skin Tests
From your past medical history, any foods that might be suspected of causing allergic reactions would be included in the panel used for skin testing. Although a valuable resource, the results are not 100 percent accurate. The tests involve putting small amounts of particular foods, which are suspected as allergens, on the skin and then scratching or piercing the skin to visually check for swelling or itching reactions.

Food Elimination Diets
The process of trying food elimination diets involves removing one

or more suspected foods from the patient's diet for about 14 days before testing to see if the food(s) are the cause. If all the symptoms are gone during that test period, the suspected allergens are then brought back into the diet, slowly, in tiny quantities. Once it is determined whether these increasing amounts cause an allergic reaction, a food regimen can be determined.

Over 35 years ago, a San Antonio clinic put people who had rather extensive food allergy responses on a tough discipline, beginning with a cleanse, fasting, then adding brown rice, with a mild vegetable broth, and herbal teas. Then other foods, one by one, were added until a reaction occurred. Once a reaction occurred, that food was removed from their diet, and others added until all allergens were determined, and a food protocol was established.

This can be a bit tough for some patients, and the clinic no longer exists. However, in theory, it is the best way to determine what foods cause an allergic reaction. The theory behind it was that once all of the suspect foods have been reviewed, the ones that are causing reactions might be avoided.

RAST Testing (Radioallergosorbent)
If you have concerns about food allergies, your physician may prescribe RAST tests for you. They involve mixing minute amounts of your blood with extracts of the suspected foods in test tubes. If it is really an allergy, your blood will produce antibodies to that specific protein, and that is easily detected. The RAST is used only to indicate allergies and not the extent of any sensitivity to those foods.

Double-Blind, Placebo-Controlled
Food Challenge Tests (DBPCF)
Here, a suspected allergen such as fish, shellfish, soy, milk, is either encapsulated or masked within a prepared item of food whereby

the patient eats it with clinical observation, checking for a reaction. This allows physicians who are trained in allergies and intolerances to determine which foods and food components cause the reaction.

Food Sensitivities

A new type of food adverse reactions used in clinical practice more recently is "food sensitivities." The body creates non-IgE antibodies against certain foods and these antibodies/food particles deposit in different parts of the body causing symptoms like joint pain, weight gain, migraine, non-allergic rashes and many others. Food sensitivities can be tested by specific IgG levels against those foods or by measuring the change in size or "swelling" of white blood cells when exposed to foods in the lab. Some manufactures of these tests call the reaction an "intolerance."

How to Prevent Allergic Reactions

The only proven method is to remove the allergen from the diet. With food intolerances, as opposed to allergies, limiting consumption to very small portions may work to avoid reactions. If you read the ingredients on food labels, knowing which foods cause allergic reactions or intolerances, and avoid that ingredient, which is the best way to avoid problems.

When eating out, at restaurants or with family or friends, ask the chef or cook about ingredients and cooking methods. That will save much grief. If the cook is offended, just explain your situation. Anaphylactic shock may be avoided especially if you are sensitive to nuts or shellfish. When in doubt, stick to grilled beef and veggies, and always carry some safe foods with you. Be prepared for any emergency, and if you have a reaction, call 911 and get help.

5. Hormone Imbalances

Perhaps it is in the area of endocrinology (after antibiotics) that modern Pharmacology has made its largest contribution. The discovery and mass production of life-saving hormones like insulin to treat Diabetes and Human Growth Hormone for Dwarfism have changed the course of medicine. Hormone Replacement Therapy for children still falls under Pediatric Endocrinologists, but more and more pediatricians are incorporating Functional Medicine concepts into their practice so that these endocrine abnormalities can be treated with a wider approach.

In the case of adults, beyond Diabetes and Thyroid Diseases treated by Endocrinologists, the most age-related decline in hormone production is managed by Anti-Aging and Functional Medicine practitioners. Still a very sensitive topic within the conventional medicine community, although in recent years there has been a wider acceptance of this practice since more research and clinical experience have accumulated.

Our bodies have an amazing system that communicates between cells, organs, glands, and all the rest. When it is all working in harmony, our bodies will maintain a sense of homeostasis and physical well-being.

The system transfers signals from the brain to the nervous system to every cell, organ, and gland in the body. This is not a one-way communication system; our body communicates with every cell inside itself. It receives messages from external stimuli, forwarding them using the nervous system, to every cell, muscle, organ, and gland, in the body. Messages come from the brain to the body, and from every cell in the body back to the brain, and from external sensations through our five senses.

It is called the neuro-endocrine-immune system. Internal and external sensations are relayed using a chemical courier system, which searches for cell receptors to transmit their messages. If the signals go astray, or are misread or not received, the cells of the body get confused.

An analogy: opening your laptop to write to your best friend on Skype to meet you for a free lunch at your favorite restaurant — but if your friend isn't online to answer, there will not be a lunch date. Therefore, your friend does not get the message that you are going to buy lunch today.

Hormones are your body's chemical courier system. They send messages to and from every system in your body. By doing this, they initiate and synchronize all functions of your body. If a hormone imbalance takes place, every bodily system is impacted. This indicates that the cause of the disease is a hormonal imbalance.

Our endocrine systems are our body's first level of delivering messages and controlling and managing the functions of our bodies. They work in harmony with our nervous, immune, and reproductive systems, as well as with the liver, kidneys, stomach and intestines, pancreas and the body's fatty tissues to coordinate the maintenance and operation of:

- Reproduction
- Growth and development
- Energy levels
- Homeostasis, the internal balance of body systems
- How we respond to our environment, stress, and injury (fight/flight response)

The meaning of the word "hormone" is Greek, meaning to set in motion, excite, or stimulate. The brain is the starting point of a hormone stimulus. The endocrine system manages the hormones of the body. It is controlled through a delicate balance, whose base is circadian rhythms. The famous expression 'biological clock' is real. It is based on circadian rhythms that influence our mental, physical, and emotional fluctuations that roughly work on a 24-hour cycle.

Most people have no idea that their endocrine system is the motor behind their biological clock. Technically speaking, external impulses of the circadian rhythm go into the body using the pineal gland. Then, they trek to every other organ in your endocrine system through the hormones. Medical science is aware that imbalance or disruption of our circadian rhythms can often lead to infertility.

Imbalances in our bodies due to hormones are common. This happens for many reasons including environment, circumstances in life, and emotions. This occurs in adults and children. It is not only an issue in middle age. Children are impacted right now more than they've ever been before as a result of environmental changes. Here are some of the hidden roots of hormonal imbalances, although there are many more.

Several Things That May Cause Hormone Imbalances:

- Chemicals found in makeup
- Chemicals we inhale from the air we breathe
- Chemicals or plastics used in packaging and production of food
- Drugs — Pharmaceutical and controlled substances
- Emotions
- Foods processed with sugar and additives
- Genetic metabolism errors
- Heavy metal toxicity
- Hormones and chemicals in the water we drink
- Hormones in meat, fowl, and chicken production/ processing
- Stress

Remember, one hormone impacts other hormones. Nutrients can impact hormone production and can benefit in hormone usage. As an example, iodine is beneficial, and fluoride from fluoridated tap water can replace iodine for the thyroid molecule. So, fluoridated water that you might consume might create an imbalance in your thyroid glands due to variation in your thyroid molecule creating differences in how your thyroid binds with other molecules. Science continues to evolve, showing us that several sub-tests of thyroid exams must be accomplished to know exactly what imbalance is present.

Once corrections are made to balance the thyroid glands, it might not be needed to control or redirect any other hormones in the body. It is really much more complex that this, but as each patient's individual history and environmental circumstances are evaluated, it's easier to identify what changes to make and explain how Functional Medicine will assist them in reaching their specific goals. Two of the hormones that must be addressed in the early stages of treatment are cortisol (adrenal gland production) and insulin (pancreatic production). Cortisol is evaluated through a saliva test while insulin requires a blood test, to test for thyroid production.

With Functional Medicine, recommendations are specific to each patient, and normally this involves nutritional guidance plus an exercise program that works for the patient.

Look at the list below — you might have hormonal balance challenges that you need to deal with. Some symptoms include:

- Allergies
- Asthma
- Autoimmune diseases
- Breast cancer or sensitivity/tenderness
- Cervical Dysplasia (abnormal cell growth)
- Cold feeling in the extremities, symptomatic of thyroid dysfunction

- Copper excess
- Depression or Anxiety
- Dryness of the eyes
- Early menstruation onset
- Fatigue symptoms
- Fibrocystic breasts
- Foggy thinking (brain fog)
- Gallbladder disorders
- Hair Loss
- Headaches
- Hypoglycemia
- Increased blood clotting (having blood clots)
- Infertility
- Irregularity with menstrual periods
- Irritability and anger
- Loss of sex drive (loss of libido)
- Memory loss (forgetfulness)
- Mood swings
- Osteoporosis (poor bone density)
- Polycystic ovaries
- Premature aging
- Skin reaction: hives, rashes, etc.
- Sinus congestion
- Trouble sleeping
- Uterine cancer
- Weight gain or Loss

Micro-nutrition is the Answer

Restoration of the hormonal balance is accomplished through the use of broad spectrum micronutrients, which include vitamins and minerals. Also, included might be amino acids and enzymes for optimum function of the body so that communication normalizes in the front lobe. Once healthy messages are sent to the hormones, communicating with the endocrine, immune, and other body systems, homeostasis starts taking place, and optimal function of the brain returns naturally. Gone are the pharmaceuticals that mask symptoms forever.

Nutrition is the primary method of treatment, and if needed, medication or supplements it temporarily needs. The brain is the seat of hormone production; it is considered the biggest endocrine gland your body has. Micronutrients help the body improve communication, through hormones, by conveying chemical signals via neuro-hormones through our central nervous system. This is an intricate pathway carrying vitamins and minerals, and also amino acids and essential fatty acids for our personal well-being. Signals then leave the brain and travel to all endocrine glands around the body (thyroid, adrenals, testicles, ovaries, pancreas) where end hormones are made. These hormones then travel to the organs where they perform their specific functions.

Taking vitamins at "recommended daily levels" really means taking the minimal amounts of micronutrients the body needs. However, if there are emotional, mental, or physical conditions that have been long-term in nature, increasing the levels of micronutrients is mandatory, and levels will vary from patient to patient.

The soil, our fruits and vegetables grow in, has virtually been depleted of minerals and other nutrients, which means our source of nutrition from plants is also depleted. Therefore, we cannot get sufficient micronutrients from our food and we are starting to require larger supplementation of micronutrients to strengthen our bodies and immune systems.

This especially applies to women who have PMS, or PPD (postpartum depression). This occurs because the newly delivered baby has literally, for nine months, sucked dry the mother's reserve of micronutrients. Doctors of Functional Medicine have discovered that mood disorders are caused, in part, by nutritional deficiencies, and that is because our food no longer has sustainable levels of vital micronutrients, or the person has an in-born abnormality to process certain nutrients and these accumulate or in other cases are depleted. This also impacts the brain's ability to function properly.

Pre-menopausal/menopausal women are especially at risk. When they've reached their mid-40s to 50s. Nutritional reserves are usually dwindling severely, and endocrine glands are not synchronized with the hormonal communication system, therefore negatively impacting all bodily systems.

Imbalance of the Male Hormonal System

Symptoms of aging in men are usually from growth hormone and testosterone declination. Once a male reaches age 20, the growth hormone has fallen and continues to fall at a median of 1.4 percent each year. By 40, men lose about half their growth hormones. Moreover, by age 80, they only have five percent of their original growth hormones. Imbalances can occur at any age. There are, however, treatment options.

Signals of Hormone Imbalance in Men

Male hormonal problems are gradual; symptoms may not seem to be important until suddenly it does not work anymore. It may seem bad one day, and good the next, but as you age, they become apparent until it disappears, or there's almost no erection at all.

Here are some symptoms to consider with erectile dysfunction:

- Anxiety
- Bone Loss (Osteopenia or Osteoporosis)
- Depression
- Fatigue/lack of energy
- Gynecomastia (growing breasts)
- Hair loss or baldness
- Heart palpitations
- Increased body fat
- Irritability
- Libido decreasing
- Memory loss (brain fog)
- Mood swings
- Muscle loss or weakness
- Night sweats or hot flashes
- Sleep apnea or insomnia

Men sometimes like to think, "I am just getting old." However, in reality, men have fathered children into their 80s and 90s. It is not aging that is the problem; it is an imbalance of hormones with aging signals. Hormone depletion and hormone imbalance are easily resolved. Through proper care, symptoms disappear and virility and normalcy return. You'll even think you are younger and healthier — because you'll certainly feel young again.

Hormone Myths in Men

There are several myths regarding hormones in aging men. The most common one is the idea that testosterone replacement therapy is a cause of prostate cancer. That has been refuted scientifically in the last few years. Not only it is safe to use testosterone in aging men, it might even be protective against acquiring prostate cancer. Even patients with previous and current (non-invasive) prostate cancer can safely receive testosterone.

Another myth is that female hormones have no role in men's health. Estrogens and Progesterone are very important in men, definitely not as important as in women, but they have their roles and a proper balance (not too much or not too little) is also important to feel well.

Female Hormone Issues

Even though rare in childhood and adolescence, female hormone imbalances start to become more prevalent in the young adult years and definitely after 40. The most common complaints I see in those years are menstrual irregularities, migraines, and PMS (Premenstrual Syndrome). Most of these complaints disappear, by the way, with general measures like the ones described in this book addressing diet, lifestyle, exercise and vitamins/nutrients supplementation and bio-identical (identical to the missing hormone) Hormone Replacement Therapy.

The Hormone Imbalance Epidemic:

Over the last 10 years, I have noticed in my practice, more and more female patients in their late 30s and early 40s complaining of hormone problems. The most common one is a lack of testosterone. Most people raise their eyebrows when I mention this since testosterone is a "male hormone." Actually, it is not the case; testosterone is also very important for the female physiology and anatomy.

Complaints related to low testosterone in women:
- Low Energy
- Mental fogginess
- Difficulty making decisions
- Lack of drive to take on new projects
- Loss of muscle definition and tone

- Higher body fat and
- Low libido and weaker orgasms

So, if you have any of these complaints, ask your doctor to check your levels of testosterone along with thyroid, DHEA, cortisol, estrogens, progesterone and some other hormones important for women.

A word about Pre-Menopause and Menopause

Considered a normal physiologic process in the life of a woman, the decline of female hormone production and the cessation of the periods is called menopause. However, many years before that (as much as 15 years according to some research) the hormones start to change, and signs of that decline start to show. We already mentioned the signs of low testosterone, but the other hormones play an important role in other functions.

Signs of Pre-Menopause:
- Menstrual irregularities
- Worsening (or improvement) of PMS
- Mood changes, especially anxiety and panic attacks
- Vaginal and skin dryness
- Lower libido
- Hair thinning and loss.

Hormone Myths in Women

It is a common misconception that for women, Hormone Replacement Therapy increases the chance of breast and other cancers. This was derived from results from the Women's Health Initiative in the 1990s and into the 2000s. The hormones used in that study were not "bio-identical" hormones but chemical hormones similar but not identical to a woman's hormones. There are even studies showing that the chance of breast cancer in women who are post-menopausal can be decreased if the right type of estrogen is used as part of the therapy.

6. Toxicities

Toxicity - Good Health Involves Detoxication At the Starting Line for the Race to Good Health through Functional Medicine

For a majority of the population, detoxification means you take some pharmaceutical laxatives or something natural in pill or liquid form, and then you camp out next to the toilet all day long.
That is a veritable misconception, and it is not detoxification. It is simply colon cleansing with substances that may not be good for your colon health. It is not even close to a solution for cleansing your body of toxins. If you do that to yourself, there are no long-term benefits whatsoever.

Functional Medicine believes that true detoxification means giving your body the support it requires to clean out toxins and impurities naturally. Detoxification helps your body work in the way that it was naturally meant to work.

Toxins are derived from two causes:
1. Internal causes, and
2. The external environment you are in.

If you do not cleanse toxins from your body, it will suffer.

Back to Basics

So, at this point, we've indicated what detox is not, let's talk about what detox is from a Functional Medicine viewpoint.

The FM viewpoint is we need to support our body's functions using the detoxification process as if it were a prescription. Look at detoxification from that viewpoint, and you are going to view it from the basic. Your body cannot be expected to work well when filled with toxins.

What Are Toxins?

Toxins exist from multiple sources. People often think that toxins are only found in the water and air. However, there are other sources including food. Not only the chemical additives in food, but the food itself, due to genetic modifications. Other hidden toxins include paints, carpets, and household cleaning chemicals, and more. Toxins are truly everywhere in our environment.

Houston is not only one of Texas' big cities, but it is the focus of the U.S. petroleum refinement industry. There are toxins around every corner. They are in the air you inhale. You cannot get away from them. Even if you are in an ideal toxin-free external environment, you still have to maintain a method of detoxifying your body. Proper detoxification is a necessary part of maintaining your health.

What is Detoxification?

Natural detoxification is not a guarantee because it can become very sluggish. This is where Functional Medicine comes in handy. Detoxification theoretically implies a natural bodily process for a specific period to eliminate the buildup of internal toxic waste. It makes an assumption that when the process is completed, the body is clean of all accumulated toxins.

Realistically, this is not how detoxification happens. Natural detoxification is all about making a fat-soluble substance into a water soluble one, for easier egestion. Egestion is defined as getting rid of undigested or toxic waste from within a cell or organ. It happens every day and depends on having sufficient nutrients available, specifically in the vitamin B family, amino acids, and antioxidants. Thyroid dysfunction, hormonal issues, and poor sleep habits hinder detoxification, amongothers.

Detoxing is a Lifestyle, Not an Event

With a poorly executed detoxification, there are normally symptoms presenting. Headaches, sexual problems, hormone imbalances are just some of them. Functional medicine is the best route to follow to realign your bodily system's functions and repair the damage caused by toxicity.

Many reasons exist for the problem. As a Functional Medicine physician, I look at the whole picture, the entire human being as a set of systems working together to make sure total detoxification takes place. If you are only viewing a single system, from a viewpoint of reducing toxification, then you are avoiding handling total detoxification of all systems - that is vital in the detoxification process. The FM approach can guide you through complete detoxification while helping you to better your life and health.

Detoxification impacts your life beyond your diet. When you use a science-based approach to detoxification, what hampers detoxification can be completely addressed. This means you can support daily detoxification, not just a short periodic detoxing process. It is a lifestyle, not something you do from time to time.

Moreover, the wonderful thing is that you will not fall for those "detox" products or schemes that claim they'll detox you. You'll be taking better care of your body and your health every day, and you'll get to a point where you will not feel the need to detoxify yourself ever. You'll be taking care of your body the way you were meant to care for it.

What is Toxicity?

Toxicity represents the extent that a substance's (poison or toxin) negativity impacts people and animals. There are harmful effects from one or more short-term exposures to toxins. Sub-chronic toxicity is when the toxic material causes a negative impact for longer than a year, but shorter than the lifetime of the person or animal affected. When a patient suffers from chronic toxicity, the toxin or combination of substances that creates the toxic effect causes harm for a very long period. This happens when there is extended exposure, usually repeated or continuous exposure, or sometimes a lifetime exposure to the toxin.

Are You a Toxic Waste Dump?

You might be if you have constant exposure to toxins, work in a chemical plant, work in a waste processing plant, work in a printing plant that still uses an ammonia processing system or any of thousands of other toxic workplaces. You should be concerned if you do.

Everyone is exposed to over a million pounds of mercury, plus billions of pounds of other toxic waste per year if we live normal lives. Just think about driving down the road inhaling the exhaust from diesel buses and trucks. It smells bad, but how it impacts the body is worse.

Thousands of chemical toxins are regularly released into our environment ever since we became an industrialized nation over 100 years ago, but most of the toxins are being released now. Sure, there are solutions with the Environmental Protection Agency, but there are constant political battles in Congress that keep the U.S. a toxic waste dump.

To clean the environment, they simply need to begin by adding scrubbers to exhaust systems in industries, cleaning their waste water, and doing a few other things. The improvements would be amazing. The big issue there is profitability of the polluting corporations. They don't want to spend a nickel of profits to have clean air to breathe for children and clean water to swim in like we did when we were children.

Ever since the onset of the Industrial Revolution, corporations are just dumping toxic waste wherever they can and wherever they think they can get away with it. Very few tests of the environment have long-term analysis, and what has been analyzed is showing some pretty unhealthy and dangerous scenarios. Perhaps that is why many companies are considering investing in setting up life on other planets to start fresh, clean lives for after we all destroy the paradise that was once Mother Earth.

Let's take a mental journey to Beijing, China for a moment. The people there are suffering from unbreathable air, and can't walk around without masks over their nose and mouth because the poison in the air is not suitable for humans to inhale. Those with respiratory or heart problems are suffering. And not only there — Mexico City, New York City, Dallas, Houston, and virtually all over the world — we are impacted by inhaling poisons. Newborn babies have been known to have as many as 287 recognized toxins in their umbilical cord blood. What does that say to you? Babies are being born into toxic futures. (Statistics, courtesy: Environmental Working Group).

If a fetus is exposed to that many toxins in the womb, how many do you think they will experience throughout their lives? If you were to go swimming in the ocean, which should be fairly clean, you will find garbage, chemical dumping, oil seepage from offshore wells, plastic from packaged drinks, cars, license plates, toilets, and human bodily waste. Can you conceive of what these poisons do to your body?

In truth, we are living in a sea of toxic waste that destroys our brains and body and makes life difficult for us to survive in and impossible for us to thrive in. Is this one of the causes of sickness and disease? Does it result in fat and obesity? I am sure that we will discover the true causes over time. Two major concepts we must realize is that we must learn how to cure diseases related to toxicity, eliminate the diseases, create a healthy homeostasis, lose weight, and build our immune system. This takes dedication to nutrition and cleansing of toxicities from the body.

The truth is, you might not learn much about toxins and detoxification from your doctor. The majority of physicians are not educated in these areas. Since nutrition and detoxification are the most important factors in treatment, you would think that medical schools would have a focus on teaching about them. This is not the case; acute care is the gold standard for treatment. Because of this, toxins and detoxification have largely been ignored by the allopathic medical field.

Because scientists and Functional Medicine physicians realize the importance of recognizing this issue, new studies are being done to help physicians learn more about it. However, there are a multitude of things that you could do yourself to reduce toxic exposure in your life. This includes enhancing your detoxification process.

Lack of detoxification is one cause of illness. So, let me begin by going over a step-by-step method you can use to improve detoxification and improve your health. Firstly, most people do not know they have any symptoms that would indicate chronic toxicity, so let's help you learn about them. If you suffer from any of the common symptoms on the list below, detoxifying yourself is probably crucial for you to begin, so you can be healthy and feel healthy again:

- Acne
- Bad breath
- Bloating
- Canker sores
- Constipation
- Diarrhea
- Difficulty concentrating
- Eczema
- Excessive sinus problems
- Fatigue
- Food cravings
- Foul-smelling stools
- Headaches
- Heartburn
- Gas
- Joint pain
- Muscle aches
- Menstrual disorders
- Postnasal drip
- Premenstrual syndrome
- Psoriasis
- Puffy, dark circles under the eyes
- Rashes
- Sinus congestion
- Skin problems
- Sleep problems
- Trouble losing weight
- Water retention

When we talk about detox, one might imagine an alcohol or narcotic detox center, or if you are more into natural and holistic, perhaps enemas or colonics. That is not what detoxification is about. Detoxification is a science relating to how our bodies eliminate waste. When waste products build up in our bodies, we become ill. The solution is to strengthen the body's ability to get rid of toxins and eliminate waste products while reducing any further ingestion of the causative poisons.

This knowledge is vital, since a majority of our illnesses that people get today are related to exposure to toxicity. You do not need to live near a toxic waste dump to get sick. It can happen from something as simple as installing new carpet in your apartment or home. Here's a list of illnesses related to toxic exposure:

- Alzheimer's disease
- Arthritis
- Attention deficit disorder
- Autism
- Autoimmune disease
- Dementia
- Digestive diseases like Crohn's disease, ulcers, and colitis
- Cancer
- Chronic fatigue syndrome
- Depression and other mood disorders
- Fibromyalgia
- Food allergies
- Heart disease
- Insomnia
- Menstrual problems like heavy bleeding, cramps, PMS, menopausal symptoms, mood changes, and hot flashes
- Parkinson's disease

With this long list, you might think that everyone has toxin-related disorders. This actually might be true to some extent. However, on the other hand, it is a relatively easy solved problem to remove toxins from your body and reduce or eliminate symptoms. In the simplest terms: "If you feel like crap, you are probably toxic."

Detoxification problems are the cause of illness, and when you investigate you'll probably find one of your body's systems needs help so you can feel and be healthy. Understanding why we are toxic and how we might detoxify ourselves is vital in getting to the point where we actually can detoxify and feel good again.

Let me first talk about something called "toxic overload." However, to do that you first need to understand what "total load" really is. It refers to the amount of all stress factors on body, at a given time. Imagine that you have a glass and you are filling it with water. Fill it to a certain point and you are at maximum load. However, when you are adding more, the water overflows, and the glass is overloaded.

When our detoxification abilities get stressed, they become overwhelmed and overloaded. At that point, symptoms come to light, and then we become ill. Yes, it might take weeks, months, or years to get sick, but that all depends on your health and the level of stress, or toxins in your body. These are a few factors that may increase your toxic load:

- Consuming a typical American food regime
- Exposure to heavy metals like mercury and lead
- Exposure to fertilizers, pesticides, petrochemicals, residues, etc.
- Food and environmental allergies, mold and toxins from molds
- Internal toxins — bacteria, fungi, yeast growing inside our intestines, and hormonal or metabolic toxins that we must eliminate
- Mental, emotional, and spiritual toxins — these include: loneliness, anger, jealousy, envy, greed, and

- hostility, all translated into toxins in our bodies
- Pharmaceutical medications, illegal controlled substances, and excess alcohol consumption can translate into toxins

Certainly, we might have the need for medications, but realistically we are a very overmedicated society, and the medication, although usually great for symptomatic treatment has secondary effects that are toxic. There exists, better ways to solve the problem; this includes changing diet and lifestyle. That is a truckload of toxins for our systems to try to expel. Therefore, you might ask — How come we are not all ill with this overload of toxicity?

That is easy. Every human being is a biochemically and genetically unique individual. Many of us have great ability at expelling toxins from our bodies, while some of us do not. Even some inherited or genetic diseases do not mean you inherited the gene that directly causes the disease but the gene that encodes a detoxification pathway for a specific toxin. Then the detoxification for that toxic substance is impaired, it accumulates and causes symptoms of a certain disease.

What Causes a Toxic Burden to Our Bodies?

Chemicals that are toxic in nature, whether they are natural or man-made often enter the human body: through inhalation, through contaminated food or water, or on rare occasions from skin exposure. A pregnant woman may pass this toxic burden to her unborn child via the placenta. Body burden means that the total quantity of this chemistry is present in your body at any given moment. Take for example lead or mercury exposure due to paint or an unsafe work environment. Some of these chemicals or their byproducts stay within us for a short time before we expel them, but if the exposure to them is long-term, it creates a persistent burden.

Let's say you have some minor exposure to arsenic or dioxin, and the body excretes the chemicals in a short period. However, if you are in an environment where these chemicals are ever-present, it then builds up and can result in death. Many chemicals cannot be excreted and are stored in blood, fat tissue, semen, bone, muscles, organs of the body, even the brain. Chlorinated products and pesticides like DDT can be stored for up to 50 years and impact your health.

Whether these chemicals are just taking a quick 72-hour trip through your body, or are stored for longer periods of time, testing can show you what your chemical load is, and designate what your daily chemical exposure is. Nearly 100,000 different chemicals are in use today in the U.S. and we've got no clue how many of them become integrated with our chemical burden. Certainly, we know many of these have already been discovered in humans globally. Scientists say the average human being now carries several hundred contaminates in their bodies — and most have not been studied.

Whether we live on an island paradise, or within a large city near a chemical factory with toxic air, dust in the air, and particulates of chemicals bind and travel a far distance from where they are created, and you get exposed. So, in a simple phrase — the big blue marble is polluted, like bathing in a chemically-based soup. Our bodies live in this polluted environment and can't help but absorb these toxins, and sometimes we store them for years and years. No matter where we are on planet Earth, we all are receptors of industrial chemicals and other toxins. So much for the saying "better living through chemistry."

Now, let's talk about pesticides. About 45 years ago, a friend of mine was taking a week-long road trip from Texas to Honduras — a week-long trip. Due to the agricultural laws in Mexico, Guatemala, and Honduras, several times on the trip, as they entered different states, their car was power-sprayed with the newest pesticide, to make sure bugs didn't go from state to state or country to country. They essentially got hosed down with DDT. The impact was strong, and they had to make frequent hotel stops to rest and drink purified water, and they still felt impacted when they returned to the U.S. some four months later. My friend feels that his health was impacted for far longer.

A variety of consumer products are impacted by the pesticides used in growing the various fruits and vegetables that later get processed into food. Dioxins and furans are produced without knowledge of what they do to the final product in the industrial process of refining and producing food. These processes include chlorine in the manufacturing and sealing of plastics used to package plastic junk food. Scientists currently feel that other byproducts are unintentionally created, which haven't even been discovered because no tests are available to identify their byproducts.

What? Have I Experienced This Exposure?

We have all been exposed to various toxins and chemicals in what we consume, water and other liquids we drink or bathe in, the air we breathe, and more. Chemicals exist on the dust particles that we tend to touch inadvertently and inhale. Dust is almost always contaminated, and it is a way that children get exposed because they are always putting their fingers into their mouths when they are very young.

Just think about what happens at the self-service gas pumps when all those petrochemical fumes escape from the gas hose as it feeds gasoline into our tanks. Moreover, what about the impact of glue, paints, dry-cleaned clothing with toxic chemicals, and what's in cosmetics, plastic food bags or boxes, home and garden bug killers? Better living through chemistry? I doubt that very much.

The life we live includes chemical cleaners for the house, bathroom deodorizers, cosmetic chemicals, chemicals in our shaving cream, even in our whipped cream. Everything has been impacted except organics that are indeed difficult to find. All chemicals in our environment sooner or later enter our body through inhalation, consumption, or skin. It is a scary world — not like the world our grandparents lived in. Moreover, it is certainly not easy to figure out the exposure, because there are so many chemicals. When you put furniture polish on your dining table and spray the air with a deodorizing spray – you make a new chemical compound that perhaps no one knows the effect of.

We do not have a food or chemical label on our bodies to show us what's in us. Perhaps, in our high-tech world, Apple or Samsung will develop a wrist watch that, through your sweat, can analyze what's going on inside you. But not today. Did you know that dioxin is found in the human body? Its presence there is from eating food — well, not organic food for certain, but it could have come from virtually anywhere.

About 75 years ago, major agricultural growers were using DDT, which was sprayed on crops by crop dusters to control the growth of various agricultural insects and mosquitoes. However, it was banned by the government in the mid-1960s because it accumulated in the fat of animals and sterilized them. Since then, dioxin has been the king of bug killers. Dioxin is no gift to mankind. It enters in various ways: herbicides sprayed on plants, and it is used in the preparation of bleached sulfite paper. Any paper you touch transfers minute amount of sulfite into your body.

No matter how it got there; it does enter the food chain making its way into what you eat. If the school or church you go to is sprayed for bugs, that is another source. Whether you live in the U.S. or elsewhere, your food supply is being impacted. Dioxin affects hormones, the reproductive system and causes cancers according to a World Health Organization report.

Pregnant mothers have another thing to worry about. Exposure to these chemicals is a heavy burden for mothers. They can attract these toxins through food, air, water, and touch. And, while they are pregnant, their babies get a dose of it as well. Chemicals in a mother's body transfer to the fetus through the placenta, which can harm the baby.

Chemicals in the mother's body also travel into the breasts and the lactation process. Chemicals transfer from the breast milk to our babies. Although mother's milk is always the best source of nutrition for babies to build their immune system, we must do our best not to be exposed to toxic chemicals during pregnancy. Breast milk still is the best source of nutrition due to its nutritional, immunological, and psychological benefits. However, industrial chemicals can get inside your infant– through contamination of breast milk and can cause problems for their development. This is something no mother wants.

Science and agriculture have known for over 100 years that chemicals can transfer into our bodies and impact health. For about 60 years, they've known this causes health problems. They have been able to measure and analyze the impact to humans and wildlife, and how these chemicals relate to health problems. Over the years analyzing methodologies have improved considerably.

Chemicals, now, have also been found in the tissues of humans and wildlife. For many years now, the government has known that some chemicals have been found in the foods we eat, the makeup people put on their faces, and in our air, and in our water supply. These studies checked fat tissues, mother's milk, semen, blood and urine and have found all kinds of chemical influences.

The Effects of Chemicals on All of Life

Chemicals impact people and wildlife differently for many reasons:
- quantity
- how long the exposure has lasted
- mode of exposure
- chemical properties

Sometimes the chemicals simply kill or damage cellular structures. Some damage the genetic material of a cell's nucleus, directly impacting our DNA and causing genetic effects that are passed on to our children. Gene mutations from food consumption can lead to cancer, reproductive disorders, and birth defects. Cancer-causing chemicals, or carcinogens, begin to act and show in tests in a matter of months. Teratogens are chemicals which are the cause of birth defects in children.

Chemicals can negatively affect reproductive ability, fetuses, and children. And these are reproductive toxins. Chemicals can damage hormone function and are endocrine disruptors. Toxic chemicals are responsible for many diseases and often can result in damage to these organs, or death:

- Blood
- Bones
- Brain
- Kidney
- Liver
- Lungs
- Nervous system
- Reproductive system

If you are old enough to remember Love Canal, or the movie Erin Brockovich, you might recall the diseases that the sufferers got from chemically-tainted water. Hundreds of diseases can come from chemical or heavy metal exposure. These include:

- Asthma
- Attention deficit disorder
- Cancer
- Depletion of breast milk
- Drop in IQ
- Endometriosis
- Hypertension
- Immune system dysfunction
- Infertility
- Learning disabilities
- Malformed genitalia
- Memory loss
- Parkinson's
- Peripheral nerve damage

Dioxin negatively impacts the development of fetuses exposed to it. Fetal exposure to PCBs causes behavioral and cognitive challenges. DDT makes women unable to generate enough mother's milk. Children's immunological abilities in some parts of the world cannot manufacture sufficient antibodies to make vaccinations effective. Fetuses exposed to mercury can develop ADD and learning problems. Fetuses and infants exposed to lead, develop brain growth impairment.

Of the nearly 100,000 chemicals used in industries, only a tiny amount of them have ever been tested for potential health impact on fetuses, infants, children, or adults. The costs of studies and tests eat into the profits of corporations; therefore, testing is only done when severe cases present, or when seeking FDA approval for the use of the chemical in the pharmaceutical industry. Even if testing is accomplished, there is no testing for what a combination of chemicals would do to anyone.

In reality, no human is only exposed to one chemical. It is more like a stew with many ingredients. Those ingredients interact, causing health problems that, at this point, no one can predict.

There is some good news (not that much) and some bad news regarding chemical testing. The good news indicates that when tests are found damaging, public interventions have often resulted in prevention from public use and reduction of exposure, lowering the body's burden. One example is that lead has been removed from gasoline and paint, and there has been a decline of lead in the human body burden in the US. Since lead causes problems with learning and intelligence in children who've been exposed, the reduction is a very positive sign.

Here's the bad news: children are still at risk from impaired function of their brains due to lead. Old housing and industrial facilities still have lead paint in some cities, and even the dirt that they plant gardens in is still contaminated. PCBs and dioxin still present problems to the public.

Epidemiology studies disease rates and causes and patterns of disease among groups of humans. It does not tell us specific chemical causes of disease or how chemicals impact health. Studies in Epidemiology virtually never can succeed in giving us primary prevention, which is the reduction of our exposure to chemicals in our environment. This is because epidemiology really doesn't have the ability to identify any specific chemical that causes disease.

Therefore, there can be no definite proof of a connection between any toxic chemical and any disease. Of course, laboratory and wildlife data can be used to create predictions regarding impact on humans. The predictions are verified by infertility, birth defects in humans, and developmental problem statistics, and certain cancer growth rates.

What About Me and My Toxicity Burden?

There is no easy way to know what the impact is on you. Even if you could discover the specifics of your personal body burden, the data might not help you. Your physician cannot prescribe medication to lower the chemical levels in your body. However, discovering your community's chemical influences might help residents to lower their exposure to toxic chemicals.

Health care facilities, laboratories, and U.S. government agencies don't provide body burden tests or evaluations. The information we have comes from very few tests of highly contaminated areas like in Pennsylvania where fracking has ruined their water supplies, and no other tests are done. What we do know is from very limited U.S. government agencies like the EPA. This comes from limited studies and only when extensive pressure is put on the agencies, and only through the threat of lawsuits, to discover why people are getting cancer or other ghastly diseases in high percentages. Studies usually analyze by age, race and gender and provide only limited information.

The studies that were done only check out a few contaminants that people are exposed to on virtually a daily basis. Realistically, you can find out more about the chemicals in beef, chicken, shrimp, lobster, other fish, turkey, and octopus than you can find out about the toxic chemicals in your own body.
One country that cares about monitoring toxic chemical burdens in the body is Sweden. They analyze and help people reduce burdens.

We have the right to know what is released into our water, our air, our food, our soil, and in all the things we consume or touch. For our own health and safety, we need to develop methods to pressure the government to perform these tests on the companies that produce our food and dirty our air. Imagine how wonderful our world would be if those in power took all the misused money and used it instead for health, education, and helping people.

Body Burden Tests

If we each were able to accomplish body burden tests, we could know ourselves better and what chemical exposure we've faced. Then, we might find a path out of the chemical nightmare most of us have been impacted with. But to date, no such thing exists — and it should be a priority to help us find a way to improve our health. Still, community-based testing helps us understand the world we live in and what can be done to improve our conditions of life.

Chemicals In our Bodies
Push Them Out, Shove Them Out, Way Out

Prevention is the most effective tool, and to do that we must eliminate the dangerous chemicals in our foods, cosmetics, water, and elsewhere that cause bodily toxic buildup. Since toxins are stored mostly in the fat cells of the body, it is going to take some time to get rid of them. If they've done organ damage, it is going to take more time, and it may not work.

States like California, Oregon, and Washington have been the forerunners in establishing standards for organic food. The people who are eating a chemical-free diet usually have much lower body burdens. However, with Big Agro-industries and their powerful lobbyists in Washington DC, we know that the problem is political. And until that changes, we know the problems will not even start to go away.

A cleansing diet, exercise, drinking enough water, using hot tubs and saunas, and the use of certain herbs all help the detox pathways and are effective ways to decrease our toxic burden. Even though chelation of heavy metals, like mercury, aluminum and lead, using oral and intravenous products are effective, these treatments are still controversial.

7. Stress

What is Stress All About?

To scientists, the term "stress" cannot be defined because it is subjective in nature. If it is not definable, how could you determine what it is, what its effects are, and what to do about it? Although scientists cannot find a description of what stress is, the dictionaries of the world certainly can, and here's a summary of what they say.

Stress is best defined as a total response to environmental demands or pressures. Not only humans exhibit stress; people who own pets can tell you that it is obvious when their beloved animals are stressed out. If we can see it in our pets, how come we cannot see it in ourselves and others?

Stress was first researched in the 1950s by Canadian doctor Hans Selye. The word was used to indicate both the cause and effects of the pressures of life. "Don't stress me," and "Don't bug me, I am all stressed out." The one big disagreement among scientists, concerns defining stress in humans. They cannot determine if it is an external reaction that should be measurable in glandular secretions or skin sensitivities, or just a subjective feeling of stress, or a reaction to stress or some combination because of that.

Human stress occurs during action and reaction of environmental influence that includes people in that environment. Must we be able to live in any environment that we perceive as filled with pressure, anxiety, tension, hassle, or worry? Of course, we're expected to perform at our optimum no matter the condition, or who puts us into that condition.

In reality, stress can be perceived as something that is threatening to our sense of balance and harmony. We lose our equilibrium, our homeostasis, and we are expected to perform at our best with what would or could be imagined as having a "gun aimed at our brains." Moreover, we must behave (like good little children) no matter the situation.

Those who apply the stress and cause the states of stress, are often the bosses, the marriage partners, the lovers, our own parents and children, those we love, those we hate, politicians, the police, the prison guards, teachers, and even the doctors who work for insurance carriers. Everyone causes stress, and everyone is the receiver of stress.

Stress is threatening the well-being of every human on earth, even the poor and starving in the world — they are under stress, and their stress cannot even be perceived by much of humanity. Stress is everywhere and in everyone, and it is not going away any time soon.

There is a belief that different people with different personalities experience stress differently. Let's say that a patient with an anxiety disorder had to work at a corporate job with stress, take the subway home from work, walk through a neighborhood which has a great deal of crime to their home, and the only thing that doctors do for them is give them Valium or Xanax. Whereas, a football player under the same situation would feel no stress because he'd probably be able to take down anyone who stresses him. Do you see the difference?

Personality, physical stress, general health, and mental well-being are all factors. Stress is the most significant cause of disease in the US and probably elsewhere. A person in stress leads a life of distress, and realistically distress leads to disease (dis-ease), or a lack of ease in life. Distress causes disease. Stress causes a major amount of illness known to man.

About Hans Selye

The term "stress,", coined by Dr. Hans Selye in 1936, who called it "the non-specific response of the body to any demand for change," really lacked clear meaning. He had realized that tests on laboratory animals treated to physical and emotional stimulation (loud noises, bright lights, too much heat or cold, and frustration) exhibited diseases of stomach ulcers, lymphoid tissue shrinkage, and adrenal gland inflammation.

It did not take long to demonstrate that those persistent stressful factors would cause "change," but really lacked clear meaning. Those diseases were caused by pathogens. Of course, tubercle bacillus caused tuberculosis, anthrax bacillus caused anthrax and spirochete caused syphilis, etc. Selye proposed the opposite that different types of insults or stresses could cause the same illnesses, not only in animals but also in human beings.

THE HUMAN FUNCTION CURVE

Any definition of stress must take into consideration a positive form of stress, or what Hans Selye labeled as "eustress." Other, more simple, examples include: winning a prize in a contest or winning an election. Thus, it might be stressful to lose, but the progress forward toward the achievement is eustress. The fear and excitement of a first kiss can be stressful and eustressful at the same time. However, once successfully accomplished, it is definitely labeled as eustress. However, going to the dentist for a tooth implant or having your appendix removed in emergency surgery, are definitely stressful situations.

THE HUMAN FUNCTION CURVE

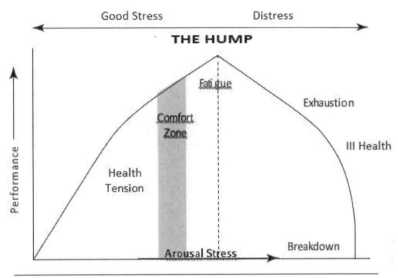

Adapted from: Nixon, P: Practioner, 1979.

Selye struggled with the definition for most of his life. When using his animal studies to try to redefine stress so people could understand what he was saying he came up with the concept of stress being "the rate of wear and tear on the body." This describes biological aging, and therefore it is not surprising that living a life of increasing stress situation will accelerate a great deal of the aging factors. One example might be premature gray hair. In his late years when asked to give a definition of stress, he said to reporters asking him, "Everyone knows what stress is, but nobody really knows."

Yes, stress is hard to define because it is different for every human being. One example is going on a roller coaster with lots of loops and flip arounds. When you observe the riders, some are pushed back in their seats, eyes closed tight, jaws clenched, hands on the safety bar, knuckles white, and screaming — that is STRESS. These stressed riders cannot wait to get to safe ground. Then there are those in the front seats, eyes wide open, seeking every possible sight of the thrill ahead for them, enjoying every second. In this example, you see some in stress and some enjoying eustress in the same activity. This means stress is also a psychological factor that varies from person to person. So, if life is a roller coaster, is your experience stress or eustress?

The use of the analogy of the roller coaster helps us to understand why the same stressor differs in impact for each of us. The riders in the rear seats of the roller coaster - were 'frightened and stressed' were so different from the ones up front who knew they had complete self-control over the ride. Neither the riders in the back screaming nor the ones up front, had any more or less control over the situation than the others, but their perceptions and fears were very different.

All too often we custom-design our stress because we have faulty perceptions of life. Moreover, as in the case of Dr. Milton Erickson, you can learn to correct those perceptions or the perceptions that others label you with. Certainly, if your life is in the back of the roller coaster, you can learn to move forward, seat by seat until you reach the front. Eleanor Roosevelt once said, "Nobody can make you feel inferior without your own conscious consent."

Although the experts can't find consensus on a definition of stress, yet with all the clinical, experimental, and personal experience that confirm the idea that we have little to no control is always distressful, learning to control it is not that difficult —and that's the other part of the story.

Effects of Uncontrolled Stress

All too often, physical and emotional disorders have their roots in stress and that includes: anxiety, depression, heart attacks, hypertension, immune system disturbances, stroke, and the weakening of the immunological system which, unfortunately, leads to susceptibility to infections, virus-linked illnesses including a common cold, all the way to herpes and AIDS, and susceptibility to certain forms of cancer, as well as other autoimmune diseases including multiple sclerosis and rheumatoid arthritis.

Stress can have a direct effect on disease of skin (hives, rashes, atopic dermatitis), and also impact the gastrointestinal system (ulcerative colitis, GERD, irritable bowel, peptic ulcer, etc.). It also is a contributor to sleep disorders, and degeneration of the nervous system with severe disease such as Parkinson's disease.

In fact, going back to that teenage boy walking into Downstate Medical school at age 14, and what he heard. It's really difficult to name any illness where stress is not only an aggravator of the situation, but more like a major player in the disease process, when not transformed psychologically into eustress (see stress effects on the body stress diagram on page 201). The list undoubtedly grows as the ramifications of stress are being determined, and the list of symptoms and diseases is forever expanding.

50 Common Signs and Symptoms of Stress
1.   Chest pain, palpitations, rapid pulse
2.   Cold or sweaty hands, feet
3.   Constant tiredness, weakness, fatigue
4.   Constipation, diarrhea, loss of control
5.   Depression, frequent or wild mood swings
6.   Difficulty breathing, frequent sighing
7.   Difficulty concentrating, racing thoughts
8.   Difficulty in making decisions
9.   Diminished sexual desire or performance
10. Dry mouth, problems swallowing food or water
11. Excess anxiety, worry, guilt, nervousness
12. Excess belching, flatulence
13. Excessive defensiveness or suspiciousness
14. Excessive gambling or impulse buying
15. Feelings of loneliness or worthlessness

16. Feeling overloaded or overwhelmed
17. Forgetfulness, disorganization, confusion
18. Frequent "allergy" attacks
19. Frequent blushing, sweating
20. Frequent colds, infections, herpes sores
21. Frequent crying spells or suicidal thoughts
22. Frequent urination
23. Frequent use of over-the-counter drugs
24. Grinding teeth
25. Heartburn, stomach pain, nausea
26. Increased smoking, alcohol or drug use
27. Increased anger, frustration, hostility
28. Increased or decreased appetite
29. Increased frustration, irritability, edginess
30. Increased number of minor accidents
31. Insomnia, nightmares, disturbing dreams
32. Lies or excuses to cover up poor work
33. Light-headedness, faintness, dizziness
34. Little interest in appearance, punctuality
35. Neck ache, back pain, muscle spasms (without injury as cause)
36. Nervous habits, fidgeting, feet tapping
37. Obsessive or compulsive behavior
38. Overreaction to petty annoyances
39. Problems in communication, sharing
40. Rapid or mumbled speech
41. Rashes, itching, hives, "goose bumps"
42. Recurrent headaches, jaw clenching or jaw pain
43. Reduced work efficiency or productivity
44. Ringing, buzzing or "popping sounds" in your ears
45. Social withdrawal and isolation
46. Stuttering
47. Sudden attacks of life threatening panic
48. Tremors, trembling of lips, hands
49. Trouble learning new information
50. Weight gain or loss without diet

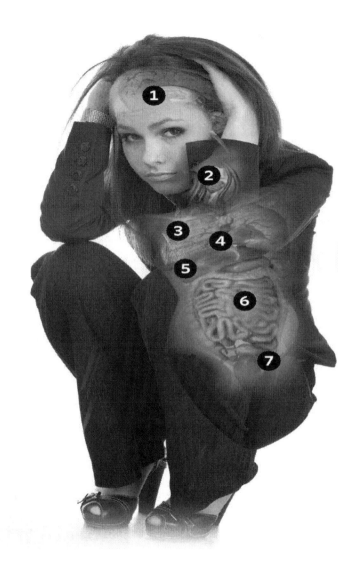

1 NERVOUS SYSTEM

When you are stressed out - whether it be physically or even psychologically - your body quickly changes its sources of energy to fight the threat that you perceive. This is what is known as the fight/flight syndrome. Your sympathetic nervous system then sends signs to your adrenals to put out adrenaline and cortisol. These two hormones cause your heart to beat rapidly, and will increase your blood pressure, slow down your digestive process, and increase levels of sugar (glucose) in your blood. After whatever crisis you've experienced has passed or gone; your body normalizes again.

2 MUSCULOSKELETAL SYSTEM

When you experience stress, all your muscles become tense. Muscle contraction for elongated periods of time cause: tension headaches, migraine-type headers, and other musculoskeletal problems.

3 RESPIRATORY SYSTEM

You breathe much harder, and can cause rapid or hyperventilated breathing which, in itself, can bring on anxiety and panic attacks for some.

4 CARDIOVASCULAR SYSTEM

When the stress is acute and for a brief period - like getting stuck in traffic with horns blowing, it causes the heart rate to accelerate and have strong muscular contractions in the heart. Dilation begins in the blood vessels which increases the blood flow to the areas that are experiencing stress. When this repeatedly happens through repetitive acute stress, it can lead to inflamed coronary arteries and a heart attack.

5 ENDOCRINE SYSTEM

Adrenals - Once your body experiences stress, your brain signals the hypothalamus, and that causes your adrenal cortex to increase production of cortisol. The adrenal medulla begins to produce epinephrine - which is often called "stress hormones." At the time that cortisol and epinephrine are released, your liver begins increasing production of glucose, which energizes the fight or flight response because your system feels that you are in a state of emergency.

6 GASTROINTESTINAL SYSTEM

Stress to your Esophagus may cause you to overeat, or to not eat enough. If you eat too much or eat foods you do not normally eat, or if you increase use of tobacco or alcohol products, you might have heartburn or even get acid reflux. Your stomach might feel the sensation of butterflies, or you may get nauseous, or feel stomach pain. If the stress is severe, you might throw up. Stress in the colon can impact how you digest food, and how your nutrients are absorbed in the intestines. You might find that severe stress causes you diarrhea or constipation.

7 REPRODUCTIVE SYSTEM

The response in men is excessive production of cortisol, produced under conditions of stress, impacting normal sexual functioning, and the entire reproductive system. Chronic stress impacts testosterone and sperm production and often results in men becoming impotent.

With women, stress in their lives can cause irregularity of the menstrual cycles, or complete absence of them, painful periods, and more. It can result in sexual desire being diminished or absent.

Workplace Stress

Study after study demonstrates that workplace stress is the number one cause of stress in American adults, and the escalation of the past few decades has indicated that it is not slowing down anytime soon. One big example is working for corporate America where one of the greatest fears of any employee is the word: "downsizing." Add to that the recent phenomena called outsourcing.

These two factors caused by selfish greed on the part of corporate management and stockholders have increased the chances of getting stress, getting sick, and dying from work-related incidents. It's like "having a bully on your back all the time with a gun aimed to your head." And, all the while you think you'll never be rewarded for all the hard work and good you have done for the company. And, "the trigger may be pulled at any time" without any cause or justification.

Many Americans during the 2007-2010 recession lost their jobs and never regained them. Some wise people began their own consulting or production businesses from their own homes. They discovered a few things:

1. You do not have to dress the part, so new wardrobes to impress the others at the office ceased to be important. Savings: thousands of dollars a year

2. They don't have to drive to work nor be seen in the newest style of clothing, newer model cars, and rarely had to meet with clients, so they didn't have higher insurance, or car payments, or time lost in traffic. Savings: thousands of dollars a year and saved transportation time

3. They do not have the cost of an expensive latte in the morning, a $20 lunch, or snacks in the

afternoon when the coffee cart comes around. Savings: thousands of dollars

4. They may have received six months to a year of unemployment compensation and sometimes a severance package that, if used properly, would help to get their business up and running, and cut their debt level down. Savings: thousands of dollars

While working at home, their health improved, the levels of stress from work decreased, and some moved to other countries where they could stay with the corporation, living in less expensive environments, learning about residing in a third world nation, and they loved the experience while keeping their jobs and benefits.

The ones who kept their jobs kept their stress, while Corporate America did them a favor, as they learned over time. After a while their stress reduced, and they didn't need a pill for this or that and fewer people experienced heart attacks after the adjustment period.

Stress Due to Job Insecurity Has Skyrocketed

- Washington Mutual Bank
- Enron
- Polaroid
- Bethlehem Steel
- DeLorean Motor Company
- World Com
- Tyco International
- Pan Am

These are a few of the companies that have tanked, sending the employees and profits into a nose dive. This has continued to happen in the U.S., and polls have indicated that 50% of the working population worries about layoffs and losing their wonderful, high paying jobs. Yes, with good reason of course. Massive downsizing and outsourcing increases investor and corporate profits and these "big boys" do not care about anything but the money. They live billionaire lives in huge untouchable mansions and pay little taxes, while those just above the poverty level are paying double the percentage of taxes.

Losing a job could put you on the streets, as homelessness increases, changing stockbrokers into beggars. Massive layoffs do not give college students hope for finding career positions when they graduate from school either.

Stress Management

> *"Stress, in addition to being itself,*
> *was also the cause of itself,*
> *and the result of itself."*
> -Hans Selye

Stress varies in everyone. There's no one size fits all solution method that reduces stress for everyone. Some people like jogging, some like aerobics, some like dance therapy and swim therapy, others prayer, meditation, self-hypnosis, chanting, tai chi, and karate. Me, I love meditation. Certainly, there are many options, including progressive relaxation (tense and release exercises), various breathing techniques, massage therapy, creative visualization, and others.

Acupressure and acupuncture, massage, Alexander Techniques, Feldenkrais, postural positioning, Reiki, biofeedback, and volunteering at nursing homes (helping others) also helps to reduce stress. Others close their eyes and listen to classical or New Age music or the sounds of nature. More recently there is humor therapy, journaling daily events, and of course playing with the dog or cat, which reduces both human and animal stress.

There are additional things such as aromatherapy, drinking chamomile or spearmint tea, drinking kava kava, taking St. John's Wort, and sleeping under a pyramid (very interesting but I don't believe any research has been completed on its effectiveness). And then there are the pharmaceutical solutions. Benzodiazepines are the best sellers.

Then come the antidepressants, hypnotic medication, and even beta-blockers used for specific issues. Additionally, there are cranio electromagnetic stimulation tools which were found safe and effective for treating anxiety, as well as mind machines for insomnia and drug-resistant depression. Group therapy, family therapy, and talking problems over with friends and family often help as well.

These are all set to work on the body and mind for the effects of stress. Yes, nothing has been really done to stop the stress. Sometimes you must realize that the application of stress in corporate situations is a way of controlling the worker so that they can get to the worker to do whatever the boss wants them to do. In the stock brokerage field, sometimes illegal activities have been forced by management on sub-management and workers have been imprisoned for doing the work that the law says is illegal. I am sure it is that way in other industries as well.

Now the focus must move to preventing stress, and that is because of the multi-billion dollar losses caused by stress. Corporations have designed courses, they teach out in nature, to relieve the stress and develop cooperation between management and the workers. But inevitably, when they return to work, within days or weeks the old behaviors of management return.

The corporations attempt to identify the sources of stress and may actually want to help reduce the stress in employees' lives. But, they rarely listen to those who are stressed to hear what they feel and see in their daily work. They already know all the answers and force solutions on workers to tell them how to reduce the impact of stress. Of course, they know it all and are the causative agent of stress — and listening and developing a rapport with workers is usually forgotten.

Instead of developing a team with a compassionate and sensitive team leadership, the boss takes the lead and tells everyone what to do and when to do it. Moreover, if there is any resistance, they destroy the team and go back to the original method of "slave driving."

We Are Responsible for Our Own Stress

We often create our stressful situations out of habits that we've formed, or our personality that has been pre-trained from childhood from seeing parental stress. This habit of creating stress can have very harmful effects as well. For example: "*My father and grandfather died of heart problems at age 51.*" I have heard this over and over, and at age 51, the patient starts feeling bad, and has some chest pain. On analysis, it's something very minor, easily remedied; but their minds are pre-set that it's a genetic fault, when it's not.

And, then there is the diagnosis — "*you have cancer and only six months to live.*" Some people have lived a dozen years by following a cognitive restructuring process with a psychologist and by working with alternative methods to modify their thought process and their behavior.

In the corporate world, time management training, assertiveness training, behavioral modification, and stress reduction methods work like an inoculation against stress. Those who don't use sound methods to gain control often begin smoking, drinking alcohol, using drugs, all to reduce stress. But, the use of these 'things' are only a solution that might work in the short-term. They really cause increased long-term stress. The long-term utilization of pharmaceutical drugs causes dependency, and over time becomes less effective and the negative secondary effects cause health problems. This can also happen with supplements interacting with each other, or with pharmaceuticals.

St. John's Wort is a long-term remedy for stress but interferes with many pharmaceutical medications. Kava kava has been banned in Great Britain. As I mentioned before, the best way to reduce stress is prevention. A good start is learning to get eight hours of sleep, and that can be had without medication, but with meditation and listening to nature sounds at bedtime. Eating a healthy diet is important, while avoiding stimulants like coffee and Coca-Cola. Take the time to learn and practice meditation — you'll find out it is wonderful to help you find inner peace.

Many people believe that their favorite stress management method works, and they have faith in it, despite the fact it may only be a placebo effect that occurs with faith in the methodology or their personal therapist.

Stress is an unavoidable part of life because virtually everything can cause stress: illness of a family member or pet, loss of your keys when you need to leave for work, or finding less money in your wallet than you thought you had. Moreover, of course, the more serious ones: divorce, death of a parent, friend, spouse, or child.

The solution is "this too shall pass." The key is learning how to devote yourself, your talents and your time to places where you are able to make a lasting difference in others' lives. That will help you find peace in your soul.

Follow the advice of the serenity prayer:

"Grant me the courage to change the things
I can change, the serenity to accept the things
I can't change, and the wisdom
to know the difference."
-Reinhold Niebuhr

Meditation for Stress Reduction

The word "meditation" often reminds me of the Hari Krishnas at the airport selling flowers, dressed in orange-colored robes. Or meeting the Sikhs, who were always doing some form of meditation, even the long-haired, heavily bearded yogis who went around the U.S. teaching about 30 years ago. That is just them. Meditation is approved by most of the medical field who have realized the benefits. To tell you the truth, meditation has tremendous value in medicine. This story comes to us from a personal experience that one of our contributors had:

"Once, in St. Petersburg, Florida I was at an acupuncture college, where they said, 'you want a clinical treatment?' I said, 'sure, why not.' First, they took my blood pressure. It was 160 over 100. They said, 'you will need many visits here, and they are $30 each but we'll, normalize your blood pressure within about a month.' I said, 'give me a few minutes alone.' I did a simple meditation and asked them to retake the blood pressure. They did — it was 135 over 85.

Immediately the director of the school walked in and said 'what's going on here'? The student explained that my blood pressure went down without treatment. The director verified it and said 'what's going on here?'

I replied, 'meditation — that is what I use to reduce my blood pressure. I thought you were going to do acupuncture for my neck pain— but when the student saw the blood pressure reading, he wanted a month of acupuncture to reduce it. I do not need that kind of help.' We talked, the director and me, and I knew two students in the class and they asked for a demonstration. I closed my eyes, there was some rapid-eye-movement (REM), I went into what's called an Alpha state and opened my eyes and said, 'DONE.' The school director was not pleased but thanked me for the demonstration, and they never got around to treating my pain in the neck. I went home and did some tense-and-release progressive muscle relaxation, took a hot shower, and wondered why people go to doctors, any doctors."

There are solutions to many forms of disease, pains, and system problems through meditation and stress management exercises. Meditation is the easiest thing in the world to do. Just put your mind at ease by controlling your focal concentration. That is all — you can direct the meditation to calm certain parts of your body, and you can add creative visualization to work on ailments you might have. You can add autosuggestions as well.

Get Comfortable

Make sure you are wearing loose-fitting clothing — no belts, bras, shoes, or jewelry, etc. You should not feel anything tight on your body. Get in a chair (straight back), or sit in a semi-lotus position, and just sit in that position in silence for a few moments.

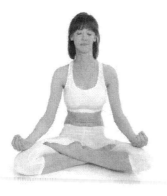 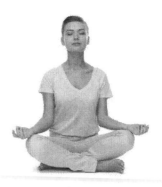

FULL LOTUS   - OR -   SEMI-LOTUS

Record this meditation and play it back to yourself, until you know how to do it automatically. Training yourself with an audio recording is highly beneficial to achieving relaxation through meditation.

"Close your eyes, and mentally check your body for tension or stress. If you notice that you have some tension in your body, just visualize it slowly melting and being replaced by a feeling of total and complete relaxation.

Begin to draw in slow, deep breaths through your nostrils. *In-In-In and hold it … and now relax and exhale.* Draw the breath in from your deepest part of your body, your abdomen. Imagine your lungs to be balloons inflating until filling up with air, and the air is coming from deep within you. *And, hold – hold – hold, and slowly exhale, imagine the balloons deflating, and you are relaxing more and more. That's right – that's good.*"

Modern Medicine for Modern Times

It's a good idea to count silently to yourself with each inhale. So, take a deep breath, from deep down inside – like from inside your stomach, and say the number ONE as you inhale and fill up your lungs. *Hold – Hold – Hold. Good, now slowly exhale.* Exhaling through slightly pursed (open) lips is the best way. *And, relax yourself.*

Now, do ten deep breaths that way, and if you wish – you can add a word at the end of the breath, like 'peace.' Personally, I like to use the word three times like this … *(exhale) … peace, peace, peace.* Say those words slowly before you draw in the next breath.

Some like to use other words, like love, balance, harmony, shalom, OM, deeper, etc. Or you can just say the word r-e-l-a-x stretched out and feel the feeling of being totally and completely relaxed.

Your focus remains on the breathing, and with each inhale, fill the lungs from deep within your stomach and feel your chest expand, and then *hold- hold-hold, and exhale … r-e-l-a-x, peace, peace, peace.*

Feel the waves of relaxation slowly moving through your body. And, in a few moments, you already feel more peaceful and relaxed. That's good.

If you ever notice that your mind has moved away from focusing on your breathing, simply let the thoughts fade away. Then gently bring your focus back to your abdomen, and the feeling of your lungs filling up. *In-in–in, hold* … and slowly exhale through your slightly parted lips, and then *r-e-l-a-x, peace, peace, peace.* That's great!

Again, scan your mind to see what thoughts and feeling you have after doing the breaths. Be aware of them, observe them, without judgment of the thoughts, or judging yourself or others; simply be an observer. Simultaneously, become aware of the changes you sense in yourself. You are changing for the better. Feel that feeling.

Do the breathing exercise for about 15 to 20 minutes. After you are finished, lie down, and relax before you get up and return to what you would normally be doing. Do this exercise once a day.

Other Forms of Meditation

Many forms of meditation exist. Here's a list for you to research and explore yourself:

- Walking Meditation
- Writing Meditation
- Eating Meditation
- Chakra Meditation
- Chanting Meditation
- Music Meditation
- Koan Meditation
- Body Awareness Meditation
- Breath Awareness Meditation
- Light/Flame/Object Meditation
- Vipisanna/Mindfulness Meditation

The Mindfulness meditation is easy. Just select a piece of fruit, perhaps like a juicy peach, or an orange, broken into wedges, or even prunes, raisins, mangoes. Draw in a few breaths, like you did before and totally relax your body. Check your body for tensions, and release them. Then, release thoughts of the past and the future. Bring your focus to the present, be open, be clear-minded, and receptive. For a minute, think about where the fruit came from. Appreciate the tree, the fruit standard, the supermarket, whatever. Draw in another deep breath and relax.

Examine the color and shape of the fruit. See it, as you have never seen this type of fruit before like you are looking at it for the first time.

Imagine the texture as you touch it, record the memory of it. Smell it and record the memory of how it smells. Take a bite, notice the juicy sweetness of it. Record the memory of it as if you have never had this flavor before. Chew it. How do you chew it? Which side of your mouth to you chew it on, the left, the right, or both sides? Become aware of that and record the memory.

Notice how many times you chew the piece of fruit before you swallow it. Don't rush, allow the sweet, juicy flavor just fill you with pleasure. Record that sensation of pleasure in your mind. Slow down, don't hurry pleasure. That's good, that's good.

If you get distracted from the meditation, just go back to the moment of eating, chewing, tasting the sweet, juicy taste, and stop; take a deep breath and then just relax. Permit the sheer pleasure of eating this fruit mindfully overtake your entire being. *Enjoy – Enjoy – Enjoy.*

Repeat this mindful meditation exercise, at least once a day, preferably before meal time. And remember, *Enjoy- Enjoy – Enjoy.* Mindfulness meditation is a truly more complex meditation, but we've simplified it for this stress management section. I suggest you study it in greater detail.

The Spiritual Side of Life

I want you to realize that there is a spiritual side to life. I do mention it to my patients, and I feel that there is a need to mention that 'we are not alone' and that there is a connection between mind, body, and spirit. Personally, I meditate, and I give thanks to this higher power for my family, my practice of Functional Medicine, and all the good that it does to help people.

One of the great successes is that a spiritual belief helps people in many ways, and they practice meditation to help them relax and find their own inner peace. Spiritual practice is an important part of life. It also works to help the Vagus nerve in your head to give you greater peace, and the ability to lose weight without stress. I strongly believe and have experienced that meditation and inner peace brings calmness and a sense of purpose in life. Yes, I try to meditate daily – you should also.

THE POWER OF INTENTION

There is something to be said about having the power of intention. The power of intention works while you speak your intention out loud to yourself. For example, *"I intend to be in control of my cravings and make good food choices for my health and well-being.* Alternatively, *"It is my intention that I shall always follow and enjoy this life-changing program and am I improving my health daily."*

CONSCIOUSNESS

"The mind, this globe of awareness,
is a starry universe that when you push off
with your foot, a thousand new roads
become clear, as you yourself do at dawn,
sailing through the light."

-Rumi

One of the processes I've learned to put to use in my life that I share with my patients is consciousness or truth, the search for a higher self. I believe it is the only answer to human suffering. I personally follow a Buddhist and Yoga lifestyle and philosophy. Even though I am not a devotee, I do my very best to follow their precepts from a modern perspective.

These perspectives include:
- Silence
- Meditation
- Contemplation
- Acceptance of everything
- Compassion
- Love

That is it. Nothing else is needed. Let's go over each of these with short discourses and quotations that should give you greater understanding of each subject. The exception is meditation (covered earlier), in which I have given you the simplest of instructions.

SILENCE

"Silence is a source of great strength."
-Lao Tzu

Silence contains an energy like no other because within it is the power to think and to act. It will slow down your mind and in that you can find inner peace.

Sadly, many people think that they need to avoid the silence with endless mind chatter, TV, or with some form of noise. Some people feel uncomfortable and alone with silence – so they use the TV for background noise so that they do not have that inner peace.

When there is silence, we turn within, and temporarily switch off ego, and refuel ourselves. Then, we begin to see the world as it should be. Often, our thoughts get in the way and we miss the beauty of life. However, when there is silence, there is openness for introspection and the opening of our consciousness. Yes, with silence we can connect to our true self which is connected to the energy around us, which in silence is pure consciousness. You can tap into this knowledge.

CONTEMPLATION

Practicing contemplation is central to being personally liberated. It is a spiritual practice that changes your state of being. Instead of being in judgment of things, it is a realization that all life is mind, thought, or spirit. Reality is truly contemplation and knowing.

The true experience of life is not possible without the concept of knowing and also living with moral discipline, while surrendering to the higher power, that dwells within you. You can accomplish that state partially through study and reading of the works of Plato, and others, and through reading, thinking about what you've read may be considered forms of contemplation.

"The contemplation of beauty
causes the soul to grow wings."
-Plato

Without surrendering yourself to contemplation, and simply living life with a goal of being healthy, wealthy or wise, genuine contemplation is difficult. This is because a moral discipline to think and discern clearly is based on a spiritual or philosophical understanding of the nature of life and reality. Therefore, contemplation with a goal of being healthy, wealthy, or wise, is not true contemplation.

"It is necessary ... for a man to go away by himself ...
to sit on a rock ... and ask, 'Who am I,
where have I been, and where am I going?"
-Carl Sandburg

Rather than following any specific goal, surrender and truly contemplate life and allow yourself to be immersed in the conscious stream of knowledge. That stream is deep within you and leads to an inner knowing through that contemplation will lead you to your own higher self and true knowledge.

"The ultimate value of life depends upon
awareness and the power of contemplation
rather than upon mere survival."
-Aristotle

ACCEPTANCE OF EVERYTHING

"Because one believes in oneself,
one doesn't try to convince others.
Because one is content with oneself,
one doesn't need others' approval.
Because one accepts oneself,
the whole world accepts him or her."
-Lao Tzu

Even though Acceptance is whole and makes no discrimination, in practical terms, I have found that if divided in three is more achievable. There are three things that need to be fully accepted, and everything else will fall into place:

Accept:
- Yourself
- Others around you
- All circumstances in life (even the negative ones provide a lesson)

Accepting others does not necessarily mean agreeing with them or not moving away from some people who are a negative force or energy. One of the greatest tragedies we experience in life is knowing that freedom is available to us, but we are trapped in the same old habits and patterns. Thus, we are entangled in a feeling of being unworthy and, we grow accustomed to living in a cage that we have created for ourselves, by our anxiety and self-judgment. Thus, we are dissatisfied with life. We become unable to access the freedom that is right in front of us, and live without inner peace, which is our true birthright.

*"Nothing brings down walls
as surely as acceptance."*
-Deepak Chopra

We may have the desire to love others without restriction, to feel true to ourselves, perhaps authentic, and to inhale the fresh air and see the beauty of nature around us. We may even want to laugh and sing, or dance to the beat of life. However, every day we, sadly, listen to our inner voice(s) that makes our life truly tiny.

Even if we are millionaires, or marry the most beautiful, if we still do not accept that we are good enough – we cannot possibly enjoy the wonderful life we've been given. Through acceptance, we can learn to see that we are restricting ourselves to a cage by our fears and beliefs. We can know that we've been wasting the precious value of life itself.

"For after all, the best thing one can do
when it is raining, is let it rain."
-Henry Wadsworth Longfellow

We can unlock the cage by accepting everything that we feel about life and our participation in it. We can accept absolutely everything, and that means be aware of what is happening in our mind and body, moment to moment, without trying to control or judge ourselves.

Instead, we have this inner acceptance of our here and now experience of life. It also means being able to feel sorrow or pain without resisting it. It also means having the desire or dislike without judging ourselves for those feelings.

"Life is a series of natural and spontaneous changes.
Don't resist them; that only creates sorrow.
Let reality be reality. Let things flow naturally forward
in whatever way, they like."
-Lao Tzu

COMPASSION

"Love and compassion are necessities, not luxuries.
Without them, humanity cannot survive."
-Dalai Lama

Buddhism teaches that to realize enlightenment, one must have two attributes: compassion and wisdom. In actuality when you have both, you can fly and see things clearly and deeply. We are taught, in Western civilization that wisdom is intellectual, and compassion is emotional, and they do not help you fly or have clarity of vision. We are even told that they may be incompatible with each other.

The truth is, Western civilization leads us to believe that emotion gets in the way of wisdom. This is in opposition to the teachings of Buddha.

"Our task must be to free ourselves
by widening our circle of compassion
to embrace all living creatures
and the whole of nature and its beauty."
-Albert Einstein

The Sanskrit word normally translated to mean "compassion" is *karuna*, which also means sympathy or being willing bear the pain that others feel. The ideal of compassion is to act selflessly to removing suffering wherever it is. Although it might be difficult, nay impossible, to eliminate all suffering, we are bound to respond despite the impossibility.

What does eliminating another's pain have to do with gaining enlightenment? It guides us to realize that the "me-me-me" concept is nothing but erroneous thought and if we are stuck with "what's in it for me?" We are not wise enough to be enlightened.

"The purpose of human life is to serve
and to show compassion
and the will to help others."
-Albert Schweitzer

LOVE

"We love life, not because we are used to living
but because we are used to loving."
-Friedrich Nietzsche

When attempting to analyze what love is we come up with several synonyms for love. Words such as acceptance, forgiveness, sharing, approving, caring, supporting, respecting. All these synonyms fall short of the true meaning of what Love is. Moreover, love must be experienced to be learned. Since love must be experienced to know its meaning and power, it is the first and foremost Earth lesson. Not taught in our public schools as part of our classroom curriculum, its lessons begin at conception and continue through life.

"God could not be everywhere,
so, he created mothers."
-Jewish Proverb

The connection between mother and child within the womb is now a commonplace discussion among women.

> *"My fetus spoke to me yesterday,"*
> *she said to her friend, "and she said that*
> *she is going to grow up to be a doctor."*

Recent research indicates that there is a connection between mother and fetus. Moreover, those mothers who lovingly educate their children while in womb, through cassette tapes, or by reading creative learning books, even listening to classical or "New Age" music, have created more loving, stable, intelligent, and healthy children.

> *"We are born of love;*
> *Love is our mother."*
> -Rumi

A Mother's Love continues throughout life. The closeness between mother and child can only be described as deep and totally unconditional love. Perhaps the same way that we, as children of a Higher Power, feel that special nurturing sense of love.

Our individual course on love continues as we grow through our family lives. It is there that we learn the intimacy of family dynamics and the beginning stages of learning. Family life is often demonstrative of what it will be like when the child matures and becomes an adult. Family life always has an environmental impact on what a child conceives of as love. Children almost always have characteristics of the parent that he or she feels closest to.

> *"Where there is love, there is life."*
> -Mahatma Gandhi

When a child goes to school, friendships are developed. This love of our friends entails high levels of respect and acceptance. These relationships with teachers and schoolmates develop into a special form of love. Friendships in school can lead to life-long friendships and even loving relationships.

"Being deeply loved by someone gives you strength,
while loving someone deeply gives you courage."
-Lao Tzu

During school and after graduation come other lessons in love. There is passionate love, such as love for a mate. This love is driven by chemistry and emotions that are extremely powerful, and enhanced by reactions in the nervous system and body chemistry.

"Love is a madman, working his wild schemes,
tearing off his clothes, running through the mountains."
-Rumi

Moreover, of course, the emotions are driven by some unknown force or power. Passion, sexuality, and the love of one another begin the cycle of the family once again. My motto is that *"Love is Always the Answer,"* to any situation, to any conflict, to any question.

"That hurt we embrace becomes joy.
Call it to your arms where it can change."
-Rumi

Spirituality

As the world continues to face challenges with religions and religious (or irreligious) warfare, we must become aware that there is a vast difference between religion and spirituality. Saying the wrong word, or using the wrong concept when talking to people, can certainly get you in trouble these days. So, we want to be clear — nothing in this book is about any religion known to man. However, this section is about having something called spirituality. Moreover, please, let us not confuse this with spiritualism, which involves talking with the dead.

*Def: **Spirituality** is the practice (like an exercise) or practical application of a process (in this case, the eight key supports) that leads to a dynamic personal transformation (permanent change) in one's life.*

Sometimes, and for some persons, it involves religious concepts, but today is more-oriented toward a subjective personal experience, and independent psychological growth. It has no connection whatsoever to any specific religious concept, and, of course, does not interfere with any religious practice.

More significantly, it can refer to a profound activity or blissful experience. As you can tell, there isn't any widely accepted definition of the concept, and it can be applied to many practices that exist today. There is more than just a definition issue here; there is an active academic difference — and these can be enlightening and helpful to you as you continue your life journey. We can look at some of the more competitive terms used to talk about this entire subject.

Faith - most people think of faith in religious/supernatural terms, such as "faith in God." Religious psychologists would label this as belief, but faith is more natural. It is from a psychological viewpoint rather than religious, and it means an innate, inborn determination in your personal search for meaning and purpose in life.

Ever since birth, everyone on earth has an innate drive that tells them there is "something more," and they want to search it down and know what's there. Just as a newborn, cries out for his mother's attention when she is no longer in sight, we as adults seek out a deeper meaning in life, a purpose in life, and significance to the question: "Why am I here?"

I know you might say not everyone is like that, but just watch the news. Today, we recognize that we live in a troubled world where people have been brainwashed, tortured, killed, and worse. This happens because we mistakenly walk into a part of the world where free thought and having faith in learning about ourselves is against the law, or the non-existence of any civil law. This is truly sad.

However, from where we are in the world, we can recognize this faith and it is a natural part of being human.
From a non-religious point of view, agnostics and atheists have this concept and this kind of faith. With religions, we hear, all too often, that "faith is a gift," and when we look at the world we see so many people without belief in a higher power. We begin to wonder if the higher power was on vacation when they were born.

In truth, everyone can enjoy the gift of faith, that inner drive to seek out and discover meaning and purpose in their lives. While it's true that some have exercised their innate gift a great deal more than others, and allow their faith to be more clearly defined and present in their lives, the question remains: Who are we to judge others?

Spirituality — some people have settled on a specific religion. Then, their spirituality is restricted to the doctrine and dogma of a specific faith in God or a church. Alternatively, they can be restricted by a belief in Mother Nature, and the practices that he or she does in life to connect with that spirituality, like prayer, doing sacraments, walking, or hiking in nature.

So, spirituality is the path a person walks, while defining their faith, as they seek meaning and purpose in their lives. Therefore, faith is an internal feeling, a consciousness that there is something more to life. At the same time, spirituality is the path we walk to discover something more in life. Spirituality occurs when your faith has been turned on. My suggestion is that you turn it on.

Belief represents your personal truths that you have deep within while you traverse the world along or at the end of your spiritual journey in life. It becomes as easier, after your spiritual quest in life, to make the decision that "this is true" and "that is not true." You, thus express personal beliefs daily that you've learned along your path of life while you've attempted to come to peace with your own inner faith. (Inner faith is every human's longing for meaning, purpose, and significance in their lives by involving themselves in spiritual practices and pursuits of their personal truths).

Religion usually refers to the particular group or community of those you share similar beliefs with, where you strive together to give support for investigating those beliefs, and making yourself and others accountable for living up to those beliefs. As a matter of reality, various religions have coded their beliefs into their sacred books, and by using rituals and their own set of moral practices, they stretch out to make a connection with deep convictions of the particular community they are in.

Feel free to use whatever expressions you feel represent how you feel in your communications with family and friends about this. These are beneficial when discussing with those who wonder about not having the gift of faith. It is helpful in understanding when someone says they are spiritual, but not religious, and many other interactions or communications that can get mired in obscurity when we use words in poorly-defined expression or hardly understood phrases.

The highest goal of any spiritual path is to surrender to it. Surrender is not a form of defeat or weakness at all. It is perhaps, the most powerful force that allows you total freedom and unlimited possibilities in life. It is trusting that the higher power, God, the Universe, or higher intelligence, can do anything and achieve anything, even when you cannot see the outcome of a challenge in advance.

Desiderata

"Go placidly amid the noise and the haste, and remember what peace there may be in silence. As far as possible, without surrender, be on good terms with all persons.

Speak your truth quietly and clearly; and listen to others, even to the dull and the ignorant; they too have their story.

Avoid loud and aggressive persons; they are vexatious to the spirit. If you compare yourself with others, you may become vain or bitter, for always there will be greater and lesser persons than yourself.

Enjoy your achievements as well as your plans. Keep interested in your own career, however humble; it is a real possession in the changing fortunes of time.

Exercise caution in your business affairs, for the world is full of trickery. But let this not blind you to what virtue there is; many persons strive for high ideals, and everywhere life is full of heroism.

Be yourself. Especially, do not feign affection. Neither be cynical about love; for in the face of all aridity and disenchantment, it is as perennial as the grass.

Take kindly the counsel of the years, gracefully surrendering the things of youth.

Nurture strength of spirit to shield you in sudden misfortune. But do not distress yourself with dark imaginings. Many fears are born of fatigue and loneliness.

Beyond a wholesome discipline, be gentle with yourself. You are a child of the universe no less than the trees and the stars; you have a right to be here.

And whether or not it is clear to you, no doubt the universe is unfolding as it should. Therefore, be at peace with God, whatever you conceive Him to be.

And whatever your labors and aspirations, in the noisy confusion of life, keep peace in your soul. With all its sham, drudgery and broken dreams, it is still a beautiful world. Be cheerful. Strive to be happy."

-Max Ehrmann,
"Desiderata" (1927)

When you are at this spiritual level, everything is always unfolding as it should. With this spiritual self, you never have to struggle or coerce anyone or situation to be the way you want it to be. The ego within you conceives that you are secluded and separate from the rest of people of your species, who are struggling to endure in the world that is hostile.

8. Physical Activity

Physical Activity - Exercise
Today's Modern World Presents Us with a Problem

Back in the time when people were hunters and gatherers, the amount of physical activity of hunting and gathering, coupled with their diet of meat and whatever they gathered, kept them strong and physically fit. However, today, most people are far less active.

Instead of hunting for food, we drive down to the local fast food drive-thru, or call 1-800-XXP-IZZA to get a delicious, but not too nutritious, pie of wheat and tomato sauce, loaded with fattening processed cheese and processed pepperoni. Moreover, it is delivered in 20 minutes to our doors. Then, our exercise is limited to lifting a slice and putting it in our mouths with some form of sugary, chemical soda to wash it down. Times have certainly changed.

Yes, the technology of the 3-minute pizza has made lives easier, but not healthier for us. Moreover, if you can see the belly fat, the unhealthy fat, like automobile tires gathering around our stomachs, and you had a way to stop this — you'd listen.

Today, we drive cars and take public transportation —buses, trains, soon even bullet trains — to get where we want to go. Walking is not considered as important to get to where we need to be. Machines do our work, wash dirty clothes and dry them out clean. We sit on couches and watch cable or satellite TV, instead of walking to the park and enjoying a walk around the lake. On TV we can see nature shows from many countries, and think we know nature.

Fewer and fewer people do manual work; robotics is taking over for our hands in factories around the United States and worldwide.

Entertainment is restricted to a large flat screen television or our laptop computer, to listening to music while we socially network with others nearby or halfway around the world.

The majority of us work in positions that involve sitting in a chair in front of a computer, or sitting on an assembly line putting together some form of advanced technological gizmo. There is so little physical effort in our work —how could we not be just a little pudgy?

As we move from our childhood to adolescence, we get gifts of cars or motor scooters, or because we have saved our money we can buy them ourselves. Everyone, from children to parents, moves their body less, burning off so much less energy and fat than we did 50 years ago.

Researchers say too many adults are sitting down for more than seven hours per day, and of course lying down to sleep. They sit at work, while traveling to work, at home in front of the TV and computer, at meals, and even on rides at theme parks.

For senior citizens, it is worse — ten hours per day sitting down, plus sleep. Senior citizens, those over 65, usually sit or lay down for 10 hours or more every day. This makes seniors, the age group of sedentary behaviors.

The Sedentary Life

The Department of Health of the United States has called inactivity the "silent killer." Sedentary behavior, like lying down or sitting, for a short period, really isn't that good for your life, health, or well-being. It is also not good for your longevity.

You must do your best to increase your activity levels, even if your bodily structure has problems doing so. You must reduce the hours that you and family members spend sitting down with screens in front of you. That being said, let's list the sedentary lifestyle behaviors to watch out for:

- being in front of a computer
- using a car for short trips when you can easily walk
- sitting down to read
- talking or listening to music while sitting

This sedentary behavior increases the risk of chronic diseases beginning and getting worse. These include:

- Weight gain and obesity
- Diabetes
- Heart disease
- Stroke

Dr. Nick Cavill (NHS, UK) has said:
"Previous generations were active more naturally through work and manual labor, but today we have to find ways of integrating activity into our daily lives...This means that each of us needs to think about increasing the types of activities that suit our lifestyle and can easily be included in our day."

Reality hits when you realize you've achieved your daily activity target, and still risk being ill with chronic health issues. This happens when you spend the rest of your day as a couch potato watching TV or lying down.

Let's give you some ideas on how to increase your physical activity and exercise in your daily life, no matter how old you are. Read for hints on increasing physical activity and increasing the amount of daily exercise, no matter what your age is; read about increasing your movement to become an active person, and do it your way. Here's where the suggestions begin.

Physical Activity

Being physically active makes you feel better about yourself, and the benefits to your health are multiplied by the energy put into each activity. An active lifestyle reduces your risk of developing:

- Heart disease
- Stroke
- Hypertension
- Some types of cancer
- Diabetes type II
- Osteoporosis

Doing a structured physical exercise program daily will assist you to lose weight and even helps reduce your stress levels. Regular physical exercise helps you to control and maintain weight, and also, to reduce stress in your life.

Brain Chemicals Are Released with Aerobic Exercise

In 1999, at Duke University, a study was done by Michael A. Babyak and James A. Blumenthal, which was printed in the *Archives of Internal Medicine*. People who exercise moderately, daily, 40 minutes, 3 to 5 days a week, had benefit. Chemicals were released into the brain. Of course, results varied among participants in the study depending on the intensity of the activity. Aerobics was performed and produced increased chemical release. The following is what the analysis of the study said about the chemicals released.

Endorphins

Endorphins, when released by the pituitary gland, occur when you are doing vigorous, sustained exercises. They are released during painful and stressful stimuli, they reduce the pain often linked with exercise, and they permit the body to exercise for longer periods of time and at increased rates of intensity. The other positive side effects include:

- Decreased stress
- Euphoric feelings (post-exercise high)
- Decreased appetite and improved immune response

Serotonin

Serotonin is a chemical released by the brain when exercising. A natural disposition booster, it reduces levels of depression. Simon N. Young, who was editor-in-chief of the "Journal of Psychiatry and Neuroscience," has indicated those with lowered serotonin often had negative effects and depression. This causes an increase in the risk of heart disorders.

Brain-Derived Neurotrophic Factor

BDNF (brain-derived neurotrophic factor) is still one more of the neurotransmitters that are released into your brain as a response to activity and exercise. This helps by reducing depression symptoms. Dr. Gary Small, in PsychologyToday.com, has indicated that it enhances brain health and improves memory.

Positive Effects of Exercise on Your Life

You can gain many positive emotional effects from exercising regularly. These positive impacts include improving your self-esteem, enhancing your mood, improving your memory and how your mind functions, and reduction of stress, thereby reducing the chance of disease. Evidence demonstrates that reduces the amount of depression in those that exercised and those using anti-depressants are very similar. More research continues.

Preferably, your goal should be 30 to 40 minutes daily of exercise at a moderately intense exercise (or at least for five days a week). Moreover, you should focus on two sessions being muscle strengthening exercise weekly, but not on consecutive days. A good goal is 30-40 minutes on the weekend and the same on Wednesday. Allow a couple of days without the muscle strengthening, so that when you build muscle you do not tax yourself beyond a certain point. Then, you let them relax for a couple of days and strengthen them again. This will build amazing muscle strength for you.

Define Physical Activity for Me, Please!

We define physical activity as some activity that has the purpose of improving and maintaining your physical condition and also improves your general overall health.

Physical activity includes three categories:

- What would be considered normal, everyday activities? Walking or bicycling to work or school five days a week. Doing deep cleaning of the house without the use of robotic cleaning devices. Working in your garden, or any type of manual labor that you may do as a part of your normal work. For example, being an automobile mechanic is a fairly active physical activity, lifting and carrying things.

- Dynamic spare time activities: i.e. dancing (this is a powerful way of being active, and stimulates the body back to be stronger). Playing with the children outdoors, or walking, or bicycling. Indoor exercise bicycles also qualify in this category.

- Sports, i.e., fitness training, aerobic dance, aerobic exercise, actively swimming (one of the best exercises because it uses almost all the muscles without great stress), and competitive sports like soccer, baseball, basketball, football, tennis, boxing, wrestling, karate — or any form of training in fitness at an exercise class.

Keeping an Active Lifestyle

The truth is that there is no guarantee of there being the perfect recipe for having great health, although the combination of eating healthy food and exercising regularly come very close to what every human being needs. Exercising regularly, or being active physically every day, benefits many systems of the body to function on an improved level. They both benefit the body by helping the body resist:

- diabetes
- glandular problems
- heart disease
- many other illnesses

The 2008 *Physical Activity Guidelines for Americans* indicates being physically active on a daily basis has the following benefits:

- Better your opportunities of having a long and healthy life
- Protects you from acquiring heart disease, stroke, or any of their precursors, like hypertension, or detrimental blood lipid patterns
- Protects you from acquiring certain cancers. The list includes colon and breast cancer, and a strong probability of protections from colon and breast cancer, and a possibly of being able to avoid cancer of the lung or uterine lining.
- Helps to avoid developing Type II Diabetes (adult onset) and also protects you from metabolic syndrome (a pattern of risk factors which increase chances of heart disease and diabetes. We'll talk more about this later).
- Reduces and prevents osteoporosis
- Lessens the risk of falling while improving senior citizens cognitive functioning
- Alleviates symptoms of depression and anxiety disorders and improves disposition
- Inhibits weight gain, and stimulates weight loss (when combined with a low-calorie diet)
- Helps with keeping the weight off after losing it
- Strengthens heart and lung tissue
- Builds muscular fitness
- Improves our ability to getting deep sleep

Inactivity Costs Everyone

Since we have enough evidence that regular physical activity and exercise are beneficial to the health of the body, you can be sure that a sedentary lifestyle does not offer benefits — it is actually a detriment. Becoming overweight and developing chronic diseases is just the beginning. Statistics have shown that only 30% of the adults in American society have reported that they do physical activities or exercise when they have enough time available. About 40% of people in the US surveyed have indicated there is no exercise whatsoever.

Studies, using special motion sensors (accelerometers) used in measuring people's activities, indicate that self-reporting of actual physical activity is not accurate. When comparing the self-reporting methods with those wearing accelerometers, it demonstrates that people are over-estimating their exercise and activity levels. The CDC indicated that lack of activity was involved in over 9,000,000 cases of heart disease, at a cost of nearly $24 billion, and this was the last available statistic from 14 years ago.

Another CDC report indicates that those having physical activities have much lower medical expenses than the people who tend to be sedentary. That being said, they got very specific, saying making people more active could reduce direct medical costs by $70 billion a year.

Can you even afford a sedentary life if you have to pay the deductible on heart problems? Being one who's labeled "couch potato" may be even more harmful because a Nurses' Health Study has found a definitive link between TV watching and obesity.

And, last but not least, researchers monitored over 50,000 middle-aged women for 6 years tracking their activity and diet. What was found was that for each 2 hours of watching TV daily, the women developed an increase of 23% chance of obesity, and 14% had an additional chance of getting diabetes. The survey indicated that it did not even matter if the females exercised or not, the more TV that they saw, the higher the risk of gaining weight and getting diabetes development. Sitting for long hours at work also seemed to have the same diabetes, and weight gain risk.

Also, studies have proven that those who are watching TV, sitting at work, and/or sitting while driving or traveling, have a much higher earlier death potential than those who are more active.

The studies tend to show that sitting for hours reduces metabolic efficiency and manages to cause severe obesity, diabetes, cardiovascular disease, and other conditions of a chronic nature.

To sum this up, take an early morning jog or a rapid walking session, or a brisk walk after lunch. Both bring a great deal of health benefits to the table. Moreover, these will not help to make up for a day of being inactive or even a day in front of the computer with the night in front of the TV. However, it will help to be more active.

So, plan your life around being active, have a regular activity/exercise routine, and remember cutting down on the time spent sitting on your butt can only help you, not hinder you.

How Much Exercise Do I Need?

If you are not a regular exerciser and don't engage in an active lifestyle daily, increasing physical activity in any way you can will benefit you. Using any aerobic activity for any length of time will increase heart rate - that is good for preventing illness. Several studies have indicated that just by walking quickly - even 1-2 hours weekly, (15-20 minutes daily) begins to lessen the potential of stroke or heart attack, or becoming diabetic, or premature death. Now, brisk walking is an undefined term, intensive walking, fast walking might be another description.

Mentioned earlier: The 2008 Physical Activity Guidelines for Americans indicates to be an adult in good health requires that you have an absolute minimum of:
- 2-1/2 hours per week of moderate-intensity aerobic activity, or
- 1-1/4 hours per week of vigorous-intensity aerobic activity,
- Alternatively, a combination of the two.

If you are not an active person, you should consider your risk of injury when starting. To reduce risk, spread out your exercise or activity over perhaps five days a week. Begin it with stretches. To combine moderate and vigorous exercise together over five days, begin by doing 20-25 minutes or so of intense aerobic exercise on two days, then about a half hour of fairly intense activity on two days.

Break it up into smaller sessions. If you can sustain the activity for a minimum of 10 minutes, you should get the benefits of the aerobic exercise for strengthening your heart and muscles.

Adults also need to do muscle-strengthening exercises at least twice during the week. On the other hand, children need at least 60 minutes or longer of an exercise that is appropriate for their age and health. This could be done with a moderate-intensity workout or swim therapy.

What's Moderate? What's Vigorous?

A moderate workout increases breathing and heart rate a little. There is a way to determine whether the activity is moderate with what's called the talk test. Physical activity must be sufficient enough for you to begin sweating, yet still you will be able to hold an almost normal conversation with anyone.

With a vigorous-intensity workout, the aerobic activity creates a far faster breathing rate with a more rapid heart rate, and you might still be able to converse — but with short sentences. Please remember that what's moderate activity or exercise for one person can be very vigorous for someone else.

A champion runner would have no problem running a mile in three minutes without stress, but his older father probably couldn't run a mile in five or six minutes without extreme stress. Think about senior citizens, they might not be able to run the mile at all unless in perfect health.

Take a Walk — or Ride Your Bike — It's fun!

It is a great gift to be able to get up and walk, and for many, it is a meditation also. Walking does not require any special equipment, just sneakers for the street or sidewalk, or even barefoot in the sand by the ocean's edge. You can walk anytime, anyplace, and unless you are in a troubled neighborhood, it is a very safe activity or exercise.

Walk slowly and it is usually no problem for most people, or you can fast walk, or race walk — and studies show that it is an exercise virtually any person can do. Numerous studies have shown that the simplicity of walking as an exercise will reduce the potential of developing cardiovascular disease, diabetes, and stroke in varying population groups.

I do not know if you have noticed, but many senior citizens do walking through parks, malls, and other places. It extends their lives and offers a myriad of health benefits, at any pace, whether brisk walking or slow walking; it is a free and easy method of exercising your body. Brisk walking, fast-walking, and race walking at three miles per hour is, of course, far more beneficial for younger people than slow walking. Fast walking is also great for weight control.

It is my observation that people who live to a very old age share three things: they walk, they eat very small portions, and they have a good sense of humor.

Cycling is Fun

As young children, we learned to ride with training wheels. Then, we graduated to two-wheelers, and then to bicycles with multiple speeds. A recent report indicates that riding a bike gives benefits similar to brisk walking. Researchers tracked over 18,000 females for more than 5 years studying relationship related to the change of their physical exercise levels as compared to their body weight. Over that time frame, the women averaged a 20-pound increase of weight during the time that the study occurred.

However, those who had the greatest exercise increase, by upping their exercise activity another 30 minutes daily, usually gained far less than those who did not vary their activity levels at all. Moreover, the type of physical activity they did also noticed a difference. Females using bicycles or did considerable amounts of walking briskly for their exercise activity could more easily control their weight. Those who walked slowly couldn't.

Walking briskly could be difficult for one person, while riding a bike maybe be more fun, and a stationary bicycle could a safer, more secure, and more comfortable alternative for losing weight. It seems that obese women walked less briskly, and for less time than women at average weight. However, when they spent the same amount of time bicycling, the impact on aerobic benefits of increasing the heartbeat and respiration was much better.

If you're not a fan of brisk walking, or riding a bicycle, any productive form of exercise like aerobic dance or swimming can make your heart beat faster and you'll breathe faster, and that will make it easier for you to meet the appropriate guidelines for activity and exercise for weight management. The only requirement is that you do it long enough and often enough to have a positive impact.

However, walking and bicycling are green activities and they are environmentally safe. They are great ways to get to work, or to a friend's house or to any event that doesn't require formal dress.

The More Active You Are, the More You Benefit

Think about this, weekly moderate-intensity aerobic activity is a great place to start. It's certainly not a recommended maximum for exercise. If you work at building a program of exercising longer, or harder, you'll bring greater health benefits to your body. Remember the caveman — every day or two, he would take his spear, a rock, and go out great distances, walking and searching, even running, to catch up with his prey and then carry it back to his cave. That usually took time, effort, and aerobic exercise. The longer and harder you work out, the better your life and health will be.

Keep in mind that your weekly minimum effort is above and beyond any light activity that's a normal part of your life. Doing fairly moderate and some vigorous activities - including dancing, swimming, and other physical activity can also be part of your total for the week if you are doing them for more than ten minutes.

Exercise Levels to Lose Weight and Maintain Your Ideal Weight

Your ideal weight can normally be found on the MALE/FEMALE weight charts, and if that is your goal, it is a fantastic experience to try to get to that point and maintain it. To reshape your body, or get rid of that change from a young and well-shaped body, and avoid "the spread" to middle age, you must watch what you eat.

There is no rule, set in stone, as to the amount of exercise needed to maintain health or improve it. But, I've been watching the performers on TV and movies, and see what they are doing. Some of them in their 50s have bodies as if they are 25-30 years old. Some will work out one to four hours daily, three to five days per week. However, their livelihood is based on looking buff and that is their choice.

So, go to a gym or use a private trainer. Some people have gym equipment in their homes, and they work hard, building a great sweat. In general, there is no set rule on how much effort and how much time is needed. You might need more than two and a half hours to feel that you've reached your ideal health goals. However, that is the starting line. When you exercise, you build serotonin, and you get a natural high from that. That is a great feeling, and it keeps your mind and body motivated to keep going, get to the ideal condition you desire and maintain it.

Begin Slowly, Increase as You Feel Good About It

The Physical Activity Guidelines for Americans, as mentioned earlier, present ideas for the population of the United States. Guidelines are not carved in stone. They are set to cover the average American, and not specifically for you.

If you've never exercised in your life, and you've been on your butt all day, sitting on a secretarial chair at work, you may need to get a little help in getting a fitness program going. Your doctor of Functional Medicine can give you a hand with that, or you can follow the guidance here.

The challenge with any guidelines established for a total country's population is that they have sought to cover the average and the majority of the population. The guidelines are not for everyone. If you are too obese to do those activity levels, you may need to adjust the guidelines. Adjustments include diet, stretches, and perhaps wearing some weights on your wrists or ankles to give you the upper hand at the outset of the program.

The amount of exercise you need depends on your genetic structure, what you eat, and your BMI. If you are carrying a great deal of fat on your frame, it is easy to give up because you might never have been exposed to an activity regime. Remember also that it depends on the size of your body, height and frame, your genetic makeup, and your ability to exercise without overdoing it.

There was a Harvard University study, 65 years ago, of about 7,000 graduates. It suggested that older and/or obese people, especially those with physical disabilities, can get as much benefit from a half hour of walking slowly, as younger people get from more intense exercise activities.

So, if you feel that a particular activity or exercise is too hard, then it might be just what you need for heart and respiratory improvement, even if it less than moderate exercise. However, if it is causing you physical pain, it probably isn't beneficial, and you should reconsider what you are doing.

Physical pain would be a sprain or strain that lasts more than a few seconds. That could occur if you are not currently active at all, and therefore, a half hour a day could be more than you can handle. Learn to gauge your progress from how you feel during and after the activity. Start out slow and build up to the 30 minutes and you'll know quickly enough. The "start slow and build up" advice has been around for a long time. It is a good form of advice for all people, but especially for seniors and the disabled.

Starting out slow will help reduce the risk of injuring yourself; and, you'll enjoy your exercise program more. If you feel your clothes getting looser, your program is successful; if you feel your clothes getting tighter, move your exercise program up a notch, and you will have no problems dropping a size or two.

Everybody, Move Your Body, Everybody, Right Now!

Have you ever noticed the hype used in advertising to get you to go to this gym, or swim club, or whatever? The ads feature hard-bodied models, of all ages, mostly young, looking great, smiling, and the opposite sex is very interested in what they see in front of them. Hype, hype, hype — it is not reality. When you think about it, the same hype goes on with smoking ads, alcohol ads, etc.

You need to prepare your mind for the reality of physical activity and exercise. If you've stopped bad habits, like smoking or drinking in excess, exercise is going to be a perfect activity for you to enjoy the feelings of being alive. Moreover, any quantity of exercises that you do will be better than nothing. The main key is to get away from your screens and do something positive to exercise aerobically for your heart and lungs. Essentially, MOVE YOUR BODY.

Better Memory Through Exercise

When you perform your moderate exercise later in life, it appears that you have a lessened risk of manifesting memory loss. A six-month program of physical exercise improves cognitive function in middle-aged and older persons. A high-intensity aerobic program improves it more and helps those who have had some memory loss.

Sadly, 10 to 15% of the people with some cognitive challenges will lose their memory function to some degree. This happens every year. This is especially sad because less than two percent of the entire nation have this problem in general. However, those who are already challenged are at greater risk. Exercise is a solution because it exercises the heart and lungs, and oxygenation of the lungs and increasing the movement of blood to your brain is an easy solution because problems go away with exercise.

What occurs is that exercise protects the body against some cognitive challenges through producing nerve-protection compounds. With the increased blood flow and the increase of development of healthy new neurons and helping the older ones survive and thrive. Thus, exercise decreases risk of heart problems and vascular disease.

Typically, when you get older, there is a strong potential for the memory and brain capabilities to deteriorate steadily with age. In the older years, you can get confused, and in the later stages be unable to take care of yourself.
However, when you keep a healthy lifestyle and dedicate yourself to your exercise and activities, this process helps you maintain good brain function throughout your life.

Studies have documented the positive impact of physical exercise on the human brain. The latest studies have documented that there are numerous positive effects that result from using physical activity and exercise in your life, and the results show that activity improves your brain function. It was determined that doing at minimum some moderate level of exercises during your 40s and 50s leads to an almost 40% decreased risk of brain impairment. The use of moderate exercise during older years indicated a more than 30% reduction of risk. Impressive results for a half hour of exercise, to say the least.

The description of mild cognitive impairment is usually a phase of transition, between the time of having a normal functioning brain, and developing problems that are more serious like Alzheimer's or dementia. Only 1-2% of the population develops dementia, and this rate might rise to 10 to 15% with those who have developed a milder cognitive issue.

The more you keep your brain active and working at its best, and can avoid cognitive impairment, the longer you'll have full brain function and the better life will be for you.

When you exercise, it pushes your brain to operate with a higher oxygenated blood flow rate, and an interesting phenomenon occurs. Oxygenation of the brain is like slowing the brainwaves down with meditation, or self-hypnosis. Once you are on that brain/mind level, what you think and what you hear have an impact on your life. If you are listening to music with words, it is important that it not be music that has bad messages in it. Often, people listen to autosuggestion mp3s, self-improvement/self-hypnosis mp3s, meditation music or nature sounds, and other things that are positive for brain and body function in the future. When you do that, your brain and mind work even harder to create the optimum for you in life.

Your Body and the Principles of Exercise

As you know, your body is an amazingly efficient machine. It is a biochemical, electromagnetic, and solar-powered biocomputer. Without the sun, your life would not last so long — that is why I say it is solar power. Imagine your body as a sleek Lamborghini for a moment. You would not let it sit in the garage, year after year, letting the oil and gas stagnate. After years of neglect, the battery will not crank, and the car will run rough if at all. Your Lamborghini needs to hit the road, be wound up and exercised.

You are your own Lamborghini, and to keep you running well, you need to change the oil (drink two to three liters of water per day), fill it with gasoline (good healthy foods proper for life), and keep moving your body. It is really simple once you get started. So, when you realize you're more valuable than any sports car, you'll take the time and the recommendations to drink water, eat healthy foods, and utilize an exercise routine incorporating one or more of these exercises:

1. **Aerobics:** Jogging, swimming, aerobic dance, elliptical machine exercises, and rapid walking are great aerobic exercises. Your heart gets pumped, oxygenation in the blood improves, you get great cellular regeneration, and more. Moreover, don't forget the increase in endorphins (natural painkillers). With exercise, life usually ceases to be a pain. Aerobics is fantastic for improving the function of your immune system.

2. **Interval (Anaerobic) Training:** Recent research has demonstrated that it is best not to walk or jog for extended periods of time. Intervals, walk 30 minutes, rest, and then walk again. It gives your heart time to start up, work out, slow down, rest, start up, work out, slow down, and rest. This is optimum for good results without putting stress on the heart or lungs. In fact, it is probably the most efficient way to burn fat. Alternate short periods of high-performance exercise with a few minutes of gentle recovery. This is called interval training and can dramatically improve your health and life. Short high-level bursts of intense exercise will help you achieve optimum health more rapidly.

3. **Strengthening:** Some people feel that they need to build their muscles with weight lifting and strength training. It is an effective program and can often produce great results like 6-pack abs.

   However, what's important is that you get with a trainer who can help you learn and build a routine of strengthening your body and optimizing the health benefits from the program. Remember, a trainer can help you avoid the mistakes that lead to strains, sprains, or other injuries.

   Repetitions can tire your body out. Do only enough repetitions so that you feel the muscles benefiting, and then STOP. Weights should be heavy enough to serve that purpose, and accomplish that goal in about 10 reps or less. Certainly, do not ever build the same muscle groups daily. They require, at minimum 48 hours to rest, repair, and rebuild themselves.

4. **Core Exercises:** There are 29 core muscles, situated mostly in your back, your abdominal cavity, and your pelvic region. These core muscles provide the strength for your body to move and to make them strong helps protect your back and spine, making them less prone to getting hurt from specific movements that aren't good for them. Building them up gives you also a sense of improved and greater stability and balance. Yoga and Pilates are excellent methods of training and building your core muscles. You can learn the proper exercises from a personal trainer.

5. **Stretching:** Not only it is important prior to start exercising, but stretching by itself is paramount for joint and ligaments health. Periodically stretching joints, neck, back in all directions and slightly beyond their limit (avoiding injuries) is useful to keep them young.

6. **Balance:** Studies have shown (and also from observing our family members and patients) that balance and stability declines with age. It is one of the first screening tests in medical offices for the aging population since it needs to be addressed to avoid falls. The older we get, the less heavy weight training and the more balance we should do. Yoga exercises are a fantastic way to maintain strength, balance, and mobility.

CHAPTER FIVE
Water and Health – No Water, No Life

"Water is the driving force of all nature."
-Leonardo da Vinci

Introduction

To be healthy mandates that we drink water. No water, no health, no life – it is that simple. Moreover, we all know that we must drink 2 liters per day and that is just a general rule of thumb – but it is for the average person who weighs about 100 to 120 pounds. A better rule of thumb is one liter for every 50 pounds of weight. So, if you weigh 200 pounds – you should be drinking about 4 liters a day.

However, no two people are alike, and no two people require the same amount of water. A person who does a triathlon requires more water, and more energy producing food, than another individual at the same weight who works in an office 5 days a week and relaxes in front of the TV set on the weekend. Activity levels, amount of exercise, the climate you live in, and your muscular condition, body fat, and more all play a part in how much water you should optimally drink.

We've discussed that the body can produce some nutrients, but one thing we know, the one essential substance we need the body cannot produce, and that is water! Because if we are not drinking enough of it, we will die. Therefore, it makes sense that water is an essential nutrient. Water is the one essential nutrient that our bodies simply can't produce on its own; we must get it from our food, or what we drink.

Because our human bodies do not have the ability to produce water, if we do not drink enough of it, we die. Therefore, it makes sense that H2O is an essential nutrient. The average human male adult is about 65% water. However, there are many factors that impact the percentage including health, weight, age, and gender. Females, on the other hand, are about 54% water. For babies, the water content can be as high as 73% in a newborn. Obese adults can be as low as 45% water. It all depends on the variable biostatistics, and that includes many factors including where you live, your race, body fat, and other factors.

The adipose (fat) in our bodies has very little water, and muscles are essentially 70% water – therefore, even though an obese person and a bodybuilder might have the same weight, their water content percentage will have a substantial difference. As we get older, we tend to lose muscle and increase our body fat – so, the amount of water we must drink, as we age, changes.

You do not need to dwell on this, but – if you are ever hospitalized and require fluids from an IV drip, you'll realize you shorted yourself over time, on your water requirements. We can maintain our muscle mass by doing resistance training, swimming, jogging, and fat levels can be kept within the norms by exerting control of our food choices while maintaining or increasing the nutritive value of food.

The Value of Water

Water enables us to quench our thirst, and it provides the body with lubrication which is vital to our good health. Vital to our health, water dissipates our heat and regulates the amount of heat lost. Imagine a radiator in a car, water (a coolant) is used to reduce the heat in the engine. It is similar with us.

Water carries our food, broken into small pieces, throughout our bodies so we can harvest the nutrients from them and transport those nutrients into our blood cells. Then, our blood carries those nutrients into every organ, gland, tissue, and everywhere that nutrients are needed.

Water is the body's essential lubricant. Water is the source of lubrication for our joints for fluid motion. The synovial fluid in our joints is made up of a high percentage of water. In addition to lubrication, water is the fluid that brings the food and nutrients throughout the body and lubricates the bowels so that it is easy to eliminate waste products.

When we cry, we release water, with a salt content. Mucous in the body is also water. Both of them are agents that cleanse the body, and remove foreign matter.

We Store Water Inside of Us

Since we are between 65 – 74% water, where is it stored? Our supply of water is mostly retained in the blood circulating in our bodies, and in the surrounding cells. Where we store it, impacts our health and balance. What we are eating, and whatever our health condition is, can change the distribution of our water. If we do not eat sufficient protein, our arterial walls can become weak, and our water might leak through into the surrounding areas. The tissues can swell, causing edema, that is water retention, and it is visible to you and your physician.

The water within our bodies is always moving, therefore, our weight is always going up and down, and that is dependent on our intake of water, and how much we eliminate. If the amount of water retained is great, or we are dehydrated, the difference can be quite significant.

Adults normally urinate about 1.5 liters per day, and through respiration, sweating, and bowel movements lose another liter. Just in case you did not know, breath is 100% water in a finely dispersed form, and when we exercise, with rapid breathing, we lose even more water. When we are sick, have fever, or diarrhea, we lose even more water. With fever and sweating we lose even more water, and can become dehydrated in the process.

The Water in Our Food

We need to stick with the guideline of 2 liters of pure, fresh, bottled water every day. If we do that, our health will improve. And do not forget there is some water in food also, so that helps. But, please don't think if you drink a liter of Coca-Cola or a pot of coffee that it can be considered water. The damage caused by sweetened, caffeinated drinks virtually destroys the water benefit in it.

In addition to those minimum 2 liters of water, your fruits and vegetables are some of the best sources of water. The usually have between 75-85% water for farm fresh or organic produce:

Watermelons	92%
Strawberries	92%
Grapefruit	91%
Cantaloupe	90%
Peaches	88%
Oranges	87%
Cranberries	87%
Raspberries	87%
Pineapple	87%

Apricots	86%
Plums	85%
Blueberries	85%
Apples	84%
Pears	84%
Cherries	81%
Grapes	81%
Bananas	74%

Fresh vegetables are also rich in water. Many vegetables have over 90 percent water content:

Cucumbers	96%
Iceberg lettuce	96%
Celery	95%
Zucchini	95%
Tomatoes	94%
Cabbage	93%
Cauliflower	92%
Sweet peppers	92%
Spinach	92%
Carrots	87%
Green peas	79%

The key word in all of this is FRESH – farm fresh, fresh organics, farmer's market fresh. Because such produce is not produced by Big Agriculture that manipulates the nutrition with chemicals.

Once veggies are taken out of the field, they begin to steadily lose their water content levels. Watermelon and lettuce have the highest water content; both have approximately 97% water content. Therefore, the consumption of vegetables and fruit is critical to us for us to keep an adequate level of water and optimal health.

Do you eat meat? Consuming lean veal is great for you because it has about 80% water, however fully grown beef only has approximately 50%.

If you require huge amounts of water, like a triathlete, and you cannot physically drink sufficient amounts to fill the need, then from your food is where you might get your extra water. Good purified, bottled water, preferable glass container, not plastic, and eating healthy fresh foods will suffice for keeping you hydrated.

Maintaining Your Balance of Fluids

Global warming, increasing temperatures literally around the world, bring heat plus humidity. These also are the factors of an environment that is significantly impacting human fluid balances, and therefore our water content, and our health. In areas of drought, high heat, like California, Arizona, New Mexico, or high humidity, like Southern Texas, Florida, Georgia people sweat more than elsewhere in the country. If you don't have air conditioning – you sweat even more.

When sweat evaporates, you feel cooler because the sweat takes away the heat. Where the humidity is always elevated, sweat will not work the same, because it does not really evaporate – and thus our cooling systems, aren't able to keep up with the demand. And the body reacts by producing greater quantities of sweat in an attempt to keep us cool. This cycle of increased sweat depletes our water supply, and simultaneously our health will be impacted if water is not replaced rapidly.

For those who live in the North, dehydration is different from sweat induced by too much heat. In the cold, we can still feel water sweating through our pores of our skin, but we may not realize the extent of the water loss and we may not rush to replace it. Sweating is the message that causes us to seek hydration through drinking water.

Do you travel by air? If you do, by traveling in a pressurized cabin at very high altitudes in an airplane, you can impact your ability to maintain water balance. Pressurized cabins have zero level of humidity.

Remember I said that breath is 100% water; when your airplane lands, the estimated humidity has gone up to perhaps 40%. Considering that our health is driven by the amount of water we have in our system, it makes sense that airplanes are incubators for diseases. So, if your flight attendant asks you if you want a bottle of water – take it. It is good for your health. And, with the tightness of airline pricing and few snack trays lately, bring money to pay for the water because it is so important to your health.

Understanding Your Hydration

Feeling thirsty? That is the last test for hydration. If you feel thirsty, you are not doing your job and thirst is not a good reaction. Drink water all throughout the day. Keep a bottle handy and sip it. Another question, what's the color of your urine on your first urination of the day? If your first urination is light yellow, kind of lighter than lemonade - you are doing good; that means your hydration is working well for you.

However, if the color is dark, like perhaps apple juice – you did not drink enough water. The solution is to grab some water, right now, and hydrate yourself. Remember 2 liters a day of purified water is the minimum amount you need to consume.

If your urine is black, purple, or red, you need to get to an emergency room right away.

Too many people think that being thirsty is a good test of hydration, but it's not – or at minimum it is really too late. There is a lag time between when we first get dehydrated and the symptoms of thirst first show up. If you are thirsty, you are already dehydrated.

The thirst mechanism in senior citizens is not as sensitive as in your people. Thus, the elderly must be aware of the fact that they should be sipping water all the time. It can become even more serious when they do not have control of their environments, like in hospitals or nursing homes. Seniors can become dehydrated because their thirst mechanism, specifically if taking medications, isn't like it was when they were in their middle-aged years. In a facility caring for the elders, extra care must be taken.

All kinds of medications, especially pain meds, can dull the senses – and the thirst mechanism for anyone taking regular pain medication is bound to be faulty. Be sure to keep up with water intake. If you are hospitalized or getting home care and have an IV saline or sugar drip – you still must drink your 2 liters of water daily. With diuretics, you'll feel thirst because the medicine is used to eliminate excess water, so the advice is still to drink water. However, your physician will better advise you on the use of diuretics and how much water to drink. Always follow your doctor's advice.

How About Salt? Should you avoid it or use it?

Salt is not as important as water since you can get your daily need from your food. But it is still very important to make sure you get your daily requirements of salt. And what do I mean by "salt"? It is definitely not "table salt." When the doctor says "Avoid eating salty foods or adding salt to your meals." He is right. But he is only right if he is referring to table salt.

Dr. David Brownstein, in his book, *Salt Your Way to Health*, explains the historical perspective of why salt was initially produced (to preserve food before canning and refrigeration were available) and how salt found its way to our tables. Most people should definitely avoid table salt since it is depleted of most of the nurturing elements, but almost everybody should benefit from using (added daily to their meals) of unrefined or "whole" salts. These are salts that are harvested from the sea or in-land mines.

It has been my personal experience with my patients that even blood pressure decreases (and some of them have actually stopped needing blood pressure medications) when they start using whole salts. An elite personal trainer even resolved a fatigue he had had for many years within 48 hours of using a whole salt. So, consider using these salts daily. If you suffer from high blood pressure, make sure you check it daily. If your blood pressure starts to rise, decrease or stop. But if it starts to drop (which is the most likely scenario), notify your physician and start decreasing (do not stop suddenly) your anti-hypertensive medications.

CHAPTER SIX
PUTTING IT ALL TOGETHER

Introduction to the Treatment of Chronic Disease with Functional Medicine

Because of the introductory nature of this book, we will briefly discuss here the most common chronic diseases that affect modern society. However, for a more in-depth discussion of these diseases we recommend our upcoming books in this Functional Medicine book series, and books from other authors mentioned in the Suggested Reading section.

Functional Medicine approaches chronic diseases in the unique way of realizing that we are indeed: body, mind, and spirit. Therefore, it is comprised of a form of medical therapy, which is in congruence of those key supports or pillars that have their independent roles but are closely interacting with one another.

Many chronic diseases have common denominators including:
- Dehydration and acidity
- Health of the gut
- Toxicities
- Vitamin deficiencies
- Inflammation
- Oxidation
- Genetic abnormalities

Moreover, other factors, which cause an imbalance in one part of the body or another. It is important to know that many symptoms and many diseases in one organ system may be a reflection a substantial imbalance in another system or part of the body.

Even if you are healthy, there are general recommendations that apply to you and everyone, whether or not there is any disease present. These recommendations are important factors that will bring your health and will keep you healthy.

Functional Medicine has the goal of preventing health challenges and taking a proactive approach to being healthy. So, when you follow these simple recommendations closely, you will avoid or delay the appearance of specific diseases in your life.

Overall recommendations to balance the eight Key Supports (pillars) will address most chronic diseases.

The 8 Key Supports are:

- Detoxification
- Vitamin Deficiencies
- Inflammation
- Intestinal Health
- Food Sensitivities
- Hormone Imbalances
- Stress Management
- Physical Activity

To begin with, it is necessary to take a dedicated level of responsibility for any chronic disease one might have, and realize that the treatment and process of curation and healing must come from the patient, and not the doctor nor the prescribed medications.
Life changes are needed so that the body can begin its healing process. So, as we begin to discuss chronic illnesses and the

protocols that are involved in their treatment, please realize that it is you – the patient, who is a primary participant in this process. We, as Functional Medicine physicians, are here to advise and support you in this process.

We will now discuss the shared root causes that affect most chronic diseases and health in general (see previous chapters for a more in-depth discussion of these "pillars"). We will then discuss specifics of the most common chronic diseases that affect modern times.

Detoxification – If you are sick with a chronic illness, there is no doubt that there is some form of toxicity in your body. There are basic guidelines to detoxification, and it is not a product that you can buy at the pharmacy, or at any health food store. It is considerably different, and detoxification is a process that goes on every day of your life.

We know that when people hear about detoxification they relate it to alcohol or drug abuse or using chlorophyll enhanced colonics. That is not the process of detoxification. What we are referring to is how the body eliminates waste from the body. We are explaining how you can better your own body's process of eliminating toxins, and also minimizing your future exposure to toxicity. This is vital because a great number of diseases are caused by toxicity of the body.

DETOXIFICATION HINTS: Detox regularly at home or supervised by a healthcare practitioner.

> **DRINK:** Plenty of water and always purified, bottled, or filtered.

> **BE INFORMED:** About environmental pollution locally (or places you travel) and be active in the community to ensure government regulations to protect the environment.

AVOID: Cigarettes (including vapor devices), side-stream smoke, alcohol, drugs, and medications unless medically necessary.

TEST: Once a year at minimum, check your body's toxic burden with laboratory tests.

Vitamins and Minerals – We all would love to think that our food contains as much of the nutrients that we need to live healthy lives. That is just not the case anymore. Why? Well, when you realize that after the *British Journal of Nutrition* reviewed 343 studies, comparing organically grown produce to Big Ag grown produce, researchers in the United States and Europe found that organic crops, and foods based on organic ingredients, had higher levels of antioxidants than conventionally produced crops.

The researchers also discovered that conventionally grown foods held higher concentrations of pesticides and a poisonous metal, cadmium. *"This shows clearly that organically grown fruits, vegetables, and grains deliver tangible nutrition and food safety benefits,"* said study coauthor Charles Benbrook, a professor of research at Washington State University's Center for Sustaining Agriculture and Natural Resources. (Source: *British Journal of Nutrition*, July 2014).

If you cannot get the nutrients from fruit and vegetables you purchase at the supermarket, it would be wise to go to the organic food produce counter or a farmer's market. The big problem is that commercially grown produce, as opposed to organic produce has toxic cadmium (a heavy metal) and numerous toxic pesticides. Moreover, we are not told about it. So, get your appropriate and healthy produce at an organic food store, or farmer's market. Also, be sure to supplement your nutrition with the following vitamins and minerals from a strong multivitamin that contains several times higher than the current RDA including:

- Vitamin D
- Omega 3/6/9
- Vitamin C
- B-Complex
- CoQ10
- Resveratrol
- Probiotics
- A strong multi-vitamin

Inflammation - plus glycation, (the uncontrolled production of protein and glucose compounds causing problems linked to diabetes and neurological conditions) and oxidation, (loss of electrons, signaling a change in the properties and charge of the molecule, which affects bonding). They are all linked to the other key supports (pillars), but there are certain actions you can take to minimize them:

> **SLEEP:** Get enough sleep, 7-8 hours a day is good for rejuvenation and rest.

> **EXERCISE:** Walk, run, swim, play sports, be active, see the exercise section for more information.

> **WATER:** Drink water. (The minimum amount of water needed is 2 liters a day, sometimes more.)

> **PLANT-BASED DIET:** Eat veggies and fruits (min. 3-4 servings per day are needed, maybe more.)

> **NO SUGAR:** Avoid excessive sugars, carbs and grains, especially highly refined products.

> **HERBS:** Use certain herbs (oregano, ginger, turmeric, cloves, Jamaican allspice, apple pie spice mixture, thyme, pumpkin pie spice mixture, marjoram, cinnamon, sage, and gourmet Italian spices.)

Intestinal Health:
Most people have no idea how important this is to a healthy life. Here're some ideas you might consider:

ANTIBIOTICS: Avoid abusing antibiotics, use if infection persists after trying all natural methods.

EAT ORGANIC: That is the best way to have healthy intestines.

AVOID: Harmful food groups: dairy, grains (especially gluten-containing grains)

AVOID: Constipation

EAT: Lots of fiber

Food Sensitivities/Foods Choices:

AVOID: Harmful food groups: dairy, grains (especially gluten-containing grains)

AVOID: Foods you are allergic to (IgE) and sensitive to (IgG), according to your trial-and-error or laboratory testing.

BE ATTENTIVE: To how you feel when eating food for the first time or re-introducing it.
Eat whole, organic foods. Incorporate super-foods like algae and mushrooms

Hormone Imbalances:

Because hormones are the body's messengers, communicating with every bodily system, they regulate all body functions. If hormone imbalance occurs, everything is impacted. Hormonal imbalance is the true cause of disease. The endocrine system is vital and must be aligned harmonically with the nervous, immune, and reproductive system, plus your kidneys, gut, liver, pancreas and your tissues to maintain and control:

- Energy levels
- Reproduction
- Growth and development
- Internal systemic balances (homeostasis)
- Stress and injury response (known as the fight/flight)

If after these general measures mentioned in this book, you still feel you have a hormone imbalance (based on the symptoms we describe in Chapter 4) have your doctor check for your hormone levels.

Cravings:

Most people crave things (I will not even call them foods) that are not good for their health. We all know what they are, and mostly they are packaged in plastic, loaded with sugar, salt, artificial colors and flavors, and other things that aren't a part of a healthy diet – and I know you think they taste good, but they are not good for you. Don't eat them – eat fresh fruit instead.

Stress:

Simply stated, stress kills. It is the force behind much of the disease and disorders of the human body and human existence. Learn to control it. My favorite method is meditation, and it is easy to learn. Practice it when you awaken in the morning, and also before you go to sleep. Be aware of the stress factors in your life, and learn to minimize them, and watch the stress disappear.

Remind yourself daily that you can be busy and going about your busy-ness, yet you can do it without having stress. If you happen to get stressed out – do some of the techniques we've mentioned in this book, convert them to eustress – and use the eustress to enable you to achieve Success.

Relaxation techniques help a great deal, so do deep breathing techniques. Consider getting help from a therapist if you do not know how to overcome stress on your own. Also, consider herbal remedies and natural stress formulas if you find that your stress levels are too hard to manage on your own.

Consciousness:
Follow the religious, faith, or spiritual path of your choice. By following these paths, you strengthen your abilities, psychologically to heal, deal with stress, to live a life with inner peace and much more. I suggest that you practice contemplation, acceptance of what is in life, having compassion, and Universal love.

Physical Activity and Exercise:
Stay active daily. Whether you are involved in an exercise program, sports, jogging, swimming, tennis or whatever – be involved. Walk rather than driving any short distance. Take the stairs rather than the elevator. Do your minimum of exercise programs a minimum of 1 ¼ hours if severe intensity exercise, or 2 ½ hours each week if it is exercise of a moderate intensity.

Vary your exercises between cardio, resistance, strengthening, core, stretching, and balance. Consider getting involved with a community program, a private gym, or a personal trainer. Take this one piece of advice to heart – move your body, be active, and remember a sedentary life is a life just waiting for health disasters to happen.

Let's move on to the treatment of specific chronic illnesses.

ALLERGIES
What Are Seasonal and Environmental Allergies?

Allergies are an overreaction, of the body's defense mechanisms, to substances that normally bring about no reaction in most people. Most of these allergic reactions are caused by allergens and bring about sneezing, wheezing, respiratory problems, and sometimes itching.

Allergies usually are not only irritating, quite a few are connected to various widespread, serious, respiratory system illnesses (like sinusitis, or asthma). Elements in your household might be the cause, and you react to hypersensitivity and symptoms, etc. Allergies may be due to seasonal changes or pollens in the air and more.

It is my strong belief (and literature on peanut and latex allergies prove) that overall allergies, and specifically the incidence of seasonal allergies, are increasing due to the facts already mentioned in this book. The reasons behind this are increasing environmental toxins, and the toxic burden on the human body, while simultaneously, our immune system competency is decreasing in these modern times.

Common Sensitivity Illnesses

- Sensitive rhinitis (also known as hay fever or "nasal," "indoor/outdoor," or "perennial" allergies)
- Insect bite/sting sensitivity: symptoms - bloating at bite, itching, and may cause anaphylaxis; can be from bees, wasps, hornets, fire ants, and yellow jackets.
- Latex Sensitivity: occurs with pure, latex rubber, those vulnerable include healthcare personnel, and may cause anaphylaxis.

- Urticaria (hives, pores and skin allergy): skin reacts, and it is typically referred to as hives.
- Atopic Dermatitis (eczema, pores and skin allergy): a frequent disease seen as skin lesions, in addition to flaking.
- Touch Dermatitis: (skin allergy): seen as skin redness; this is a frequent work disease.
- Conjunctivitis: (eye allergy): seen as redness of the eyes. Symptoms include itchy, watery eyes.

Allergies and their symptoms aren't only hay fever and watery eyes. Symptoms can also be:

- Tonsillitis/adenoid enlargement
- Headaches
- Persistent vomiting
- Runny nose
- Upper respiratory infections
- Asthma
- Wheezing
- Pneumonia
- Sinusitis
- Otitis media (ear infections)
- Nasal polyps
- Anaphylaxis
- Dermatitis
- Edema
- Pharyngitis (sore throat)
- Attention deficit disorder
- Urticaria (hives)
- Mental slowness

What Can Cause Allergies?

The substances that bring about the allergic response are called "allergens," or perhaps protein allergens like chemicals, pollen, food, or dust. Most of these substances can get into our bodies through numerous methods.

They are inhaled through the sinuses as well as the lungs. Examples are airborne pollens (connected with specific bushes), grasses and weeds, environmental toxins in the air, household dirt (with dust mites, mold spores, cat and dog dander), or latex, as well as nature (poison ivy, poison sumac, even pine, tend to be examples). Moreover, sometimes medical treatment including Penicillin, or injectable drug treatments, etc.

The capacity to develop an allergy to cat dander could be 3 to 4 long time exposures to a cat prior to demonstrating signs and symptoms. Poison ivy sensitivity (contact dermatitis) is a type of sensitivity where genetics plays no part. This reaction commonly occurs in youth from wandering in the woods. Further, chemicals in deodorants and makeup products, can also result in contact dermatitis.

Allopathic Medical Diagnosis and Treatment

Most allergies can be diagnosed in either of two ways: description of the occurrence of symptoms, or a skin test. If you go to the physician and you react with hives from the sting of a flying insect, or a symptom of sneezing and irritation to the face and head from the appearance of a cat – the diagnosis is rather easy, and so is the treatment. If what you are going through is not so obvious, and is caused by other factors, then a scratch test (at minimal) is required. Sometimes, blood tests can also be performed to find the offending agent.

Therapy depends on the results of your tests as well as the signs and symptoms you present. The obvious way to prevent an allergic reaction is to stay away from the substance you react to as much as possible, or to eliminate any substances from your home as well as other surroundings.

Treatment includes:

- Antihistamines reduce rashes and/or hives, as well as itching, sneezing, and irritated or blocked sinuses.
- Decongestant supplements are also used to reduce stuffed noses by diminishing inflamed sinus membranes.
- If vision is impacted by burning or itching, eye drops may be indicated to rid yourself of symptoms involving the eyes.
- Corticosteroid ointments, like Clobetasol, reduce irritations due to rashes.
- Corticosteroid nasal sprays are available to alleviate swelling that produces nasal congestion, not including the "rebound" consequence from non-prescription sinuses sprays.
- Cromolyn salt also stops the release of inflammatory chemicals such as histamine from mast cells.
- Epinephrine is sold in self-injectable, pre-measured doses. It is the only medication which works in the case of a life-threatening anaphylactic attack. It has to be used within a few minutes of the first symptom of a serious reaction.
- Immunotherapy (Allergy Shots and more recently Sublingual Immunotherapy (SLIT)/Allergy Treatment). If your reactivity does not clear up with the above treatments, immunotherapy might prevent allergies. Over time, the patients become less sensitive to that allergen.

Functional Medicine Approach

The Functional Medicine approach parallels the evaluation and partially parallels the allopathic method to some degree. If you are suspected of having any chronic illness, lab tests would be performed to verify or supplement what has been discovered from your medical history and physical exams. All of the data points, history, physical examinations, and laboratory tests help guide an FM physician in making decisions for treatment.

Treatment though is more multi-factorial including:

- Avoidance of the allergen or offending factor
- Boosting the immune system with vitamins/minerals, stress management, etc.
- Regulating histamine response by avoiding certain foods (cheeses, wines, canned foods).
- Consider supporting the degradation of food-derived histamine using Diamine Oxidase.
- Testing and avoiding IgG-mediated food sensitivities.
- Address adrenal (cortisol) imbalances if present.
- Correct Leaky Gut if present that might be a contributing factor.
- Consider herbal therapies (Stinging nettle and Spirulina)
- Use antihistamines or steroids only temporarily and for moderate or severe cases while the root causes are fixed.

AUTOIMMUNE DISEASES

About 8% of the U.S. population now realize that they have been impacted by an autoimmune disease. There is uncertainty regarding that figure being totally accurate because that is just diagnosed cases. The supposition is that this might be just the tip of the iceberg. Some say the total number of affected people may even be double that amount. Autoimmune diseases include:

- Addison's disease—an adrenal hormone insufficiency
- Celiac sprue disease—gluten reaction is damaging the small intestine's lining. Gluten is in barley, rye, and wheat
- Grave's disease—hyperactivity of the thyroid
- Hashimoto's disease—thyroid gland inflammation
- Inflammatory Bowel Disease (IBD) – Inflammatory diseases involving esophagus, colon, and small intestine (Crohn's Disease and Ulcerative Colitis)
- Multiple sclerosis—impacting the brain and spinal cord
- Pernicious anemia— because of inability to absorb vitamin B12 there is a reduction in red blood cell count
- Psoriasis—causes redness and irritation of the skin, with thick, flaky, silver-white patches
- Rheumatoid Arthritis—joints and surrounding tissues become inflamed and painful
- Scleroderma—a disease of the connective tissue that creates changes in the skin, muscles, blood vessels, and internal organs
- Systemic lupus erythematosus—impacts the brain, joints, skin, kidneys, and other organs
- Vitiligo—white patches on skin due to loss of the skin's pigment
- These are just a few of the major diseases of autoimmune disorders.

Autoimmune diseases impact over 25 million known sufferers, and perhaps a whole lot more. This epidemic is quite huge, albeit a quiet one, because the media does not ever report it in the news. However, still it is very real, and people are becoming permanently disabled from it – some are dying from it while suffering horribly in the process.

The cause of Autoimmune diseases is not yet known, but a good guess would indicate that it is most probably related to toxicity:

- We eat foods that are toxic
- We eat foods (and lots of it) that we might not be able to digest completely, especially gluten-containing grains.
- Heavy metals are in our environment and our foods
- Toxic chemicals exposure is an almost daily occurrence
- Long-term antibiotic usage is not the greatest thing for us either
- Moreover, the level of stress that we live with these modern times is fairly severe

These probably have resulted in severe epidemic conditions in sufferers who know about their illness, and even those who do not that they even have the problem. More people suffer from autoimmune diseases than from cancer or heart disease, and yet most people do not even understand why they are suffering and what these diseases are all about.

There is certainly a lack of knowledge about this group of illnesses. This lack of awareness results in considerable pain, disability (and deforming results) and also death, and too much of it goes either incorrectly treated or completely untreated.

People with these disorders struggle with horrible systemic issues because doctors cannot really determine what has gone wrong, and cannot therefore find any solution for their health issue. This is because medical science has not found the direct cause of their problem.

Symptoms of Autoimmune Diseases

If you are experiencing any of these symptoms, especially if it's a combination of more than one of them, you could be suffering from an autoimmune disease.

- Muscular pain, joint pain, weakness, or tremors
- Insomnia, rapid heartbeat, heat intolerance, weight loss
- Sun-sensitivity, reoccurring rashes or hives, a rash across your nose or checks shaped like a butterfly
- Difficulty in focusing or concentrating
- Weight gain, cold intolerance, feeling tired
- Loss of hair, white patches inside the mouth or on the skin
- Stomach pain, blood or mucous in the stool, ulcers in your mouth, diarrhea
- Dry skin, dry eyes, dry mouth
- Numbness/tingling of your feet or hands
- Multiple blood clots and/or miscarriages

So, the Big Question is: Why does the Immune System Attack Healthy Body Cells?

Since the actual cause(s) of autoimmune diseases has not been discovered by the medical or scientific field, at this time, we cannot answer that question. However, if you know a member of your family has any autoimmune disease, you might be likely to develop one also. Theories exist regarding the causes, and they include:

- bacteria or viruses
- drugs
- chemical irritants
- environmental irritants
- Reactive arthritis —inflammation of urethra, joints, and eyes; can create sores on skin and/or mucus membranes
- Sjögren's syndrome—destroys the tear-producing glands and saliva, thereby causing dry mouth and eyes; can also affect kidneys and/or lungs

However, no one knows for certain what the cause of autoimmune disease might be.

Although there is no known cause, conventional medicine uses long-term medications including thyroid medicines, antibiotics, anti-inflammatories, NSAIDs, steroids, etc. for treatment of these diseases. Often this results in a combination of secondary effects that are like a snowball rolling downhill.

The increasing trend of using immune modulators (like Cyclosporine, Tacrolimus and Methotrexate), even in early stages of disease, are known to have serious side effects like increased risk of scarring of the liver and lung and lymphomas (cancer of the lymphatic system).

Although there is no known cause, there is hope and positive results from the use of Functional Medicine. This is because Functional Medicine is aimed at searching, by looking within, at the different bodily systems, for potential ways to reverse the problem.

The Approach to Treating Autoimmune Diseases Through Functional Medicine

Just one example is provided here before we talk about autoimmune diseases as a group. For autoimmune thyroid problems

Hashimoto's Disease – Functional Medicine approach includes the supplying of thyroid hormone if needed, for the short-term, but it goes further. It also works toward trying to preserve the health of the thyroid gland, and the patient's health through patient's thyroid gland and health by addressing the problem of an overactive immunological system.

Traditional medical care ignores the immune system by simply replacing the thyroid hormone with only pharmaceuticals treatment for the long-term. The Functional Medicine approach includes caring for the immune system. The reason behind this is that once a patient has one autoimmune disease; others may follow including Lupus Erythematosus, Crohn's, MS, rheumatoid arthritis, and others.

Through Functional Medicine, other autoimmune disorders can be treated. The problem is not that the tissues are being attacked by the autoimmune disease, it is that that immune system is running wild. Lifestyle changes that reverse that problem make the autoimmune system tranquil, and balance in the immune system is necessary for the problems to resolve.

Suppressing the immune system when running wild will not help the situation at all. To survive life, we all require immune systems that are fully functional so that we are protected from viruses, fungus, bacteria, and to protect us from our potential of developing cancer or other diseases.

In actuality, there are probably more than 100 different autoimmune diseases, they are all chronic that are caused by the immune system. Moreover, if caught early enough, before they progress causing severe pain and disability, they are all treatable. The first sign is that fatigue, muscle, and joint pain are occurring and possibly a feeling of exhaustion. At that point, blood tests are required so that you can be properly diagnosed.

With proper changes in your lifestyle, your immune system can be normalized, achieve systemic homeostasis, and brought back into a condition of balance before any damage is irreversible.

Because the immune system is the defense for your body against invading illnesses, it's always ready to attack. Sometimes, the system gets confused and attacks you. It is often difficult to know friends from enemies and your bodily tissues sometimes are invaded in error. When your body is fighting infections or an allergen, or even a response to stress or food, somehow it makes an error in judgment and attacks you – your thyroid, stomach, skin, brain, and joints, actually it can attack everywhere.

Conventional medicine does not know how, as of yet, to discover what is causing the confusion? However, Functional Medicine can help draw a roadmap to discovering what's gone wrong, and why the immune system is attacking the wrong cells. When conventional medicine treats these problems with drugs like NSAIDs, steroids, methotrexate, it can cause kidney failure, muscle loss, osteoporosis, diabetes, depression, infection, psychosis, and far worse. All because the immune system responds to these medications as if they were foreign invaders.

However, whenever these medications are used during a short period of time, selectively, and proper lifestyle changes are put into place, they do help the users to get their lives and bodies back on track. They're never a long-term answer – they should not be considered long-term and the final goal. However, instead, they should be considered just a temporary stop gap so the immune system can take a short vacation while we are evaluating and treating the cause of the illness.

One thing to realize is that third world countries do not have autoimmune disorders, at least not at such high rates as industrialized ones. Those living there without running water, pre-prepared foods, conveniences like chemically treated food, toxic air and water, and all the other amenities of life simply don't get autoimmune disorders. Most people who grow up in the country, on a ranch or a farm, don't get these disorders either. This is because their immune systems are trained by nature to recognize what's dirty, or what's infectious, or what is an enemy (bugs, snakes, etc.) and their immune systems recognize what's good for you and what's not.

Today's automated lifestyles with toxicity everywhere, in the air, in the water, in our food, the immune system simply cannot do an advanced chemical analysis of all the things attacking it. Therefore, the confusion occurs. The Functional Medicine approach is an approach to intelligent investigation and discovery of the underlying causes, or systemic imbalances that cause chronic illnesses including autoimmune disorders.

The process of questioning the patient and examining the patient is vital. The search for toxicity and allergens, and infections – along with the common causes of inflammation, is vital. With that knowledge, the true cause of disease can be unveiled and treated. In many cases, the overuse of antibiotics has caused damage to the gut flora, the healthy bacteria, resulting in opportunistic yeast infections. Abnormal bacteria can overtake the gut because of this, thus causing leaky gut syndrome and many food sensitivities including gluten and dairy products. This is a possible cause of autoimmune diseases.

Because of the modern world, we live in, we are invaded by toxins at home, at work, while traveling, and including our air and water. As a result, we develop opportunistic infections, another possible cause of autoimmune diseases. The solution is, of course, to do a deep cleaning.

After the initial evaluation, the Functional Medicine doctor will use short-term treatments for infections with antibiotics, and short-term treatments of yeast with anti-fungal medications until the problem is gone. During that time, the immune system can take a break.

Food allergies can be dealt with appropriately and during this time the immune system rebuilds and rebalances itself. However, a lifestyle change is required to get healthy again.

This includes supporting the immune system with the use of herbs, zinc, vitamins, probiotics, and a healthy organic, whole-food, allergen free diet. Usually, that is a good part of all that's needed. At that point new lab tests are taken. When it is confirmed that all the results are normalized – you get the message that modern life can be part of the cause and conventional medicine might be the instigator through pharmaceutical overuse. How we treat our bodies to rebalance and stay healthy is often the proper treatment for autoimmune diseases.

Instead of just alleviating the symptoms with drugs, if you are suffering from an autoimmune disease, this is a good plan for you and your physician to work together to rebalance your health:

- Evaluate for infections you may not know are there — yeast, bacteria, viruses, etc. — and take note of inflammatory problems, and get them treated.
- Check for food allergens you weren't aware of with IgG and IgE food testing. Start a diet which eliminates these allergens.
- Get checked for Celiac sprue disease. It's a simple blood test, which can be done through your medical doctor.
- Check yourself out for heavy metal toxicity: Mercury and many other metals tend to wreak havoc on your immunity system resulting in autoimmune diseases.
- Get your gut in good condition, inside and out. Get checked out for Leaky Gut Syndrome.
- Get on a healthy diet, more plant based than meat based. Supplement your health with nutrients like fish oil, vitamins and minerals, and probiotics that will make your immune system more responsive and help it to achieve homeostasis.

- Exercise regularly, it is perhaps the best anti-inflammatory ever devised. Get involved in a program to be active and involved with physical activity daily as discussed in this book.
- Do yoga, meditation, deep breathing, massage, and relaxation therapies – because stress weakens the immune system, and these practices strengthen it.
- Use ancient whole or super-foods like microalgae and edible mushrooms
- Use a doctor of Functional Medicine. He or she will help you achieve your healthcare goals faster, in a more natural way, minimize the overuse of medication, and without being exposed to the toxicity of modern life. You may also bring this book or this information to the attention of your Primary Care Physician

CANCER
What is Cancer?

Cancer is a specific class of illnesses that is most often characterized by rapid abnormal cellular growth. There are more than 100 types of cancer, each classified by the name of the cell that is affected. Cancer damages the body through uncontrolled cellular division and forms masses, or lumps that are called tumors. The exception to the rule is leukemia where the normal blood function is impacted by abnormal cellular development in the blood.

Tumors develop and grow uncontrollably and interfere with all systems: circulatory, digestive, nervous system, endocrine, etc. They often release hormones, impacting the function of the human body. Tumors that remain in one location, and have limited growth, are normally labeled as benign tumors.

Malignancy

Dangerous, malignant, tumors develop when two things happen:
- A cancerous cell expands locally to adjacent tissues, destroys healthy cells in its path and disrupts those new tissues – this is called invasion.
- The cells that travel to distant organs, then divide and grow on those organs, producing new tumors – this is called Metastasis.

Treatment:
There are four major approaches to treatment of cancer:
- Surgical procedures
- Radiological therapy
- Chemotherapy
- Immunotherapy

Four goals to achieving a cure from cancer:

- Treatment
- Prevention of reoccurrence
- Prolongation of survival
- Palliative care

SURGICAL PROCEDURE

Localized cancers usually are, in the beginning stages, in only one location with a defined border and structure, and are subject to removal by surgery, with surrounding lymph nodes removed at the same time. They have minimal chance of propagation to other parts of the body. Cervical cancer can be dealt with using surgery, and often a hysterectomy is performed. Ovarian cancer is frequently diagnosed surgically. Surgical treatment may be the primary treatment and may be totally curative. Other strategies to treatment like radiation therapy or chemotherapy may be required.

THE RADIATION REMEDY

Radiation therapy is done through different procedures. Normally, radiation is used for specific localized tumors in need of treatment. The procedure usually is for a relatively small area of the body and is normally repeated every day or a few days for several sessions. The X-rays, gamma or other types of rays penetrate the body supposedly killing cancerous cells. In the process, healthy cells may also be damaged in the attempt to kill cancerous tissue.

CHEMOTHERAPY

Chemotherapy is a chemical therapy with the usual side effect of hair loss. Chemotherapy introduces anti-cancer drugs into your blood and they enter almost every area of the body Chemotherapy interferes with cell duplication. That is the theory, but healthy tissue might be impacted by chemotherapy as well. Chemotherapy includes negative secondary effects, most prominently weakening the immune system.

IMMUNOTHERAPY

Immunotherapy continues to be tested as a cure for cancer. In theory, immunotherapy may be a positive treatment for cancer because it mobilizes your body's immune system to help eliminate cancer tissue. There's a great deal of investigation being done on immunotherapy, but it is now of minor professional importance and its foundation for curing cancer is yet to be developed. This immunity process offers the body protection against illness by building antibodies that fight invading microorganisms.

INVESTIGATIONAL REMEDY

There are varied investigative research programs being done for cancer cures. Most of this research might be divided into several categories, alternate, unusual, or unconventional therapies.

Alternate or unusual treatments are labeled that way because they've never been proven to be effective. Had they been effective, it would already be a conventional treatment. To be proven effective, normally requires randomized research comparing one treatment against another.

Unconventional treatments are needed in certain situations. They give faith where there probably has never been any before. They encourage sufferers to be involved more and do more to manage their situation. At this time, options are philosophical, not medical.

Functional Medicine as a Workable Alternative

Allopathic medicine simply focuses on naming the diseases by considering their locations in the human body, along with its niche description, and defining a pathway for treatment based on the above methods.

The naming of ailments does not help the patient understand what's causing the disease, and it is an old-school method of diagnosis. The more we learn about the mysteries of our bodies, and the sciences of chemistry and biology, the more we will discover that alternative concepts work, because they fine tune the body, and each system that's out of sync.

Functional medicine doctors prefer a different way to address the disease, by determining WHY the disease occurred in the first place. What are the fundamental reasons or essentially WHY has this disease occurred? We simply look inside of us, per se, to learn what's happening with us.

Traditional allopathic medicine is like attempting to diagnose your vehicle by simply noting a particular noise it is making without ever lifting the hood and checking underneath it. Functional Medicine lets us look inside of us and discover the real causes behind it.

Looking inside of us gives us a way to figure out the particular systemic problems when an ailment comes up and shows you how to modify the situation in a more positive way.

This particular move to an increasingly well-designed, systems-based, environmentally friendly, approach seems to be one of the ways 21st-century healthcare is now being aimed. Consider cancer in a brand new light – finding the remedy by looking inside of us. The problem with the normal allopathic method is this - we are thinking about the disease in the wrong way.

This particular reality seemed to be highlighted again and again by experts in the field of cancer treatments. They essentially indicated how thinking about specific types of cancer is essentially mistaken. Simply because you put a label on a particular ailment, doesn't mean you realize what's appropriate treatment, or, for that matter inappropriate? Nor can you determine by a label how to treat everyone who has it.

Classification of tumors simply by human body site - lung, organ, breast, brain, intestines, and so on - misses the mark at locating particular fundamental reasons, or mechanisms, along with the pathways that help to develop a certain type of cancer. The fact cancer shows up at a particular place in the human body informs you of practically zero concerning why that cancer initially began. It also allows you no knowledge concerning how it began in any affected person.

Two people suffering from cancer in differing areas of the body could have produced cancer for identical reasons. Also, two different people suffering from identical types of cancer could have produced it for different reasons. An individual suffering from prostate cancer and another with intestinal cancer could have more causes in common than two sufferers of intestinal cancer. In the past, we've practiced medicine by location – in which an ailment happens in the body. That does not make sense any longer.

We now have the potential to deal with cancer by realizing the fundamental mechanisms along the metabolic pathways. Most of these, and other beliefs concerning cancer, along with its treatments are producing frightening results.

Did you know, there was a two-year survey between the years 2008-2009, where the US President's Committee determined that people had grossly underestimated the connection between what they called environmentally-friendly toxins, plastics (PETs), chemical substances, and cancer risk? They've also discovered how personal views and feelings, along with overall stress and pressure effect increased the risk of cancer. Rather than managing cancer by changing the environment holistically, we continue to use allopathic treatment to try to manage it. However, that does not work. While several people know which tumors grow slowly and gradually for many years prior to discovery, literally millions of people in the US are unknowingly developing cancer somewhere prior to diagnosis.

There is a "war" on cancer, which we are battling for a reason: we're going towards the wrong goal. We see many problems that could potentially be at cause of cancer:

- A nutrient-poor diet brimming with sugars and fats
- Insufficient exercising
- Immune imbalances
- Inflammatory imbalances
- Continual stress and pressure
- Depression
- Oxidation-reduction imbalances and mitochondropathy (disease of the cell part called mitochondria)
- Persistent pollutants
- Heavy metal toxicity
- Hormonal and neurotransmitter imbalances
- Detoxification and biotransformational imbalances
- Digestive, absorptive, and microbiological imbalances

We could shift our focus from less divisive methodology and onto much more positive views that, therefore, cause more positive emotions—which are all good fertilization for that garden within the backyard of the human body. The long run of cancer attention should use medicine's knowledge of the particular workings of ailments along with information to build physiologic and metabolic stability, to create therapies that assist us by enhancing regular physiology.

These pieces of the particular problem which have the advice for cancer prevention along with cure are scattered around the panorama of medical technology. They want simply to be built right into the history which could guide future professional medical attention. Any time will be ripe to help accelerate this procedure.

A simple outline of positive efforts toward bettering health might be:

- a nutrient-dense, plant-based diet,
- use of superfoods (microalgae, mushrooms),
- drink enough water,
- physical exercise,
- modifying views along with reactions to help the pressure, and stress
- along with detoxification

That could be a good start in getting the garden ready in the particular backyard where cancer grew up. When you take care of the garden all the plants (systems) benefit.

We can easily improve our immune system functioning by dietary changes and lifestyle changes, nutrition, and phytonutrient enhancements. Without question, we can use detoxification processes for personal cleansing to reduce the use of carcinogenic chemical substances.

We can assist in the cleansing of toxic estrogens by modulating the diet, the way of life, and by reducing hormone-disrupting xenobiotics or petrochemicals. We could also modify how our genetics are shown by modifying the factors that manage its manifestation. These include diet, vitamins, phytonutrients, toxins, stress and pressure, as well as other options for treatment of infection.

The list of positive actions is numerous. However, you get the point - there is a positive method to strengthen the immune system and probably slow down or even stop, the growth of cancer and beat it especially as an adjuvant to the conventional radiation therapy, chemotherapy, etc. Considering the outcomes of traditional allopathic treatment, isn't it time for the Modern Medicine called Functional Medicine to be used for the betterment of the patient and the medical field in general?

CARDIOVASCULAR DISEASE
What is Cardiovascular Disease?

About 625,000 people in the United States are dying annually caused by heart disease. That is essentially one out of every four people who die, die of CVD (coronary heart disease). CVD is the primary cause of death for women and men. Over half of deaths from heart disease were men.

Around 750,000 Americans have a heart attack annually. Approximately 550,000 have their first ever heart attack, and about 200,000 are having a second, or third, etc. Hypertension, elevated LDL cholesterol, and smoking are three of the main risks causing CVD. Around 50% of all Americans are exposed to at least one of these three, causing them to be at risk for cardiovascular disease. Other health conditions, as well as lifestyle choices, put Americans at risk for cardiovascular disease, and they are:

- Poor diet
- Physical inactivity
- Overweight and obesity
- Diabetes
- Excessive alcohol use

Symptoms of Cardiovascular Disease

Everyone thinks that chest pain is the one and only sign of cardiovascular disease. Conversely, not all people suffering from cardiovascular disease have chest pain. Some can even go through a heart attack without feeling any chest pain. Also, by the time they do feel pain, they probably have had cardiovascular disease like atherosclerosis for a long period of time.

There is only one way that's guaranteed to detect early, whether you have cardiovascular disease, before something serious happens and, that is through a comprehensive examination from your medical doctor, and making sure you get appropriate medical care. Symptoms of cardiovascular disease can be vague or mild and might include:

- Anxiety
- Backache
- Change in consciousness
- Chills
- Cough
- Cyanosis (blue discoloration of lips, hands, and feet)
- Dizziness
- Edema (swelling of the ankles or legs)
- Fainting
- Fatigue
- Indigestion
- Nausea
- Pain or numbness in the extremities
- Paleness
- Palpitations
- Shortness of breath
- Sweating
- Vomiting
- Weakness

In infants, the symptoms would be different including:

- Feeding difficulties
- Not gaining weight

Cardiovascular Disease Risk Factors:
- Cigarette smoking
- High blood cholesterol
- Passive smoke
- High blood pressure
- Overweight
- Obesity

Conventional medicine treatment for CVD:
- Diet changes: low salt diet
- Lifestyle changes: Exercise. Stop smoking. Limit alcohol intake.
- Pharmaceutical medications including:
  - 1. Diuretics medications
  - 2. Central Alpha 2 Adrenergic Receptor Agonists like Clonidine
  - 3. Adrenergic Inhibitors
  - 4. Beta Blockers
  - 5. ACE inhibitors
  - 6. Calcium Channel Blockers
  - 7. Vasodilators
  - 8. Postganglionic sympathetic inhibitors

Simplified summary of the FUNCTIONAL MEDICINE APPROACH for CVD:
- Note physical signs and findings which could be useful in a Functional Medicine diagnosis of the physiology and pathophysiology of CVD.
- Analyze testing to discriminate between normal and non-normal physiology which is specific to CVD and many related endocrine disorders.
- Apply understanding of lab testing to prioritize treatment for the individual patient.
- Choose the appropriate methods of treatments for CVD.

These are possible causes of hypertension leading to CV disease:

- Magnesium deficiency
- Depressed testosterone levels
- Bacterial infections
  - Strep A.
  - H. Pylori
  - Chlamydia
  - pneumonia
- Viral infections (Coxsackle virus, CMV)
- Cadmium, lead, mercury toxic exposure
- Compromise of the detoxification process
- Deficiency of Taurine
- Fatty Acid Imbalance
- Kidney dysfunction
- Antioxidant insufficiency

Functional Medicine – Diagnostic Process
First step:
1. Check patient's BP
2. Get past medical records/history from prior treating physicians.
3. Do a medical questionnaire, including pre-birth medical history, in utero history, children, adolescent years, teen years, young adult, adult, etc.
4. Perform standard laboratory tests
5. Do lab tests and review results of
   a. Blood chemistry panel: lipid and metabolic profiles
   b. CBC with differential
   c. Check CRP, Homocysteine, Fibrinogen levels
6. Advanced testing
   a. Rule out bacterial pathogens
   b. Rule out heavy metal toxicity
   c. Evaluate nutrient deficiencies

    d. Evaluate fatty acid balance

    e. Evaluate Sex Hormones

    f. Evaluate liver load

    g. Evaluate antioxidant status

7. Some of these additional tests may be required for:

    a. Lipoprotein factors and ratios

    b. Chronic inflammatory markers

    c. Ferritin

    d. Fibrinogen

    e. C-reactive protein

    f. Insulin

    g. Testosterone

    h. Sex hormone binding globulin

    i. Free androgen index

    j. Magnesium

    k. Oxidant stress factors

    l. Homocysteine

    m. Coenzyme Q10

    n. Vitamin E

    o. Lipid Peroxides

    p. Essential Amino Acids

    q. Toxic elements

    r. Fatty acids – plasma

    s. Organic acids in urine

    t. Compounds of bacterial or yeast/fungal origin

    u. Check for C pneumonia antibodies

Other things to be aware of:

- Chronic low-level lead exposure can cause hypertension and CVD or myocardial infarction and death:

- High levels of lead or mercury can indicate chronic hypertension and generalized atherosclerosis, renal dysfunction with proteinuria.

- High intake of mercury from non-fatty freshwater fish creates an accumulation of mercury and high risk of acute myocardial infarction and dying from a chronic heart disease.

- Take note: H pylori and C pneumonic infections are linked to coronary heart disease.

"Heavy metal toxicity, especially mercury and cadmium, should be evaluated in any patient with hypertension, CHD, or another vascular disease."
-Houston MC. Altern-The Health Med 2007;13 (2):s128-33.

"The association between blood lead levels and increased all cause and cardiovascular mortality was observed at a substantially lower blood lead levels than previously reported."
-Menke A, et al. Circulation 2006; 114(13):1388-94.

Functional Medicine approach might include Systemic Detoxification, plus:
- Coenzyme Q10 – CO-Q10
- Magnesium
- Potassium
- Omega 3
- Hawthorn
- Garlic

Therapeutic lifestyle change, dietary changes (with a food plan), mind, body, spirit practices including meditation, and exercise and patient education.

MENTAL AND NEUROLOGICAL DISORDERS

Your brain is the focal center of thoughts, memories, and experiences. All of them are stored in your brain. The entire higher control center of your body's entire nervous system is located there. Your ability to enjoy, understand, feel, and know what life is about is determined by how your brain functions. It's comprised of over 100 billion neuronic circuits. Each of these circuits is connected to thousands of others; so, your brain has trillions of connections. Without a healthy brain, it's impossible be a healthy personal mentally and physically.

Ask yourself a few questions:

- Do you feel the lack of drive, depressed, or mentally fatigued?
- Is your thinking foggy or unclear?
- Are you nervous or anxious, or have trouble relaxing?
- Do you struggle to remember names, locations, telephone numbers, or anything else?
- Are you having a hard time focusing and completing your tasks?
- Do you have a neurological disorder?

If your answer to any of these is "yes", you might be struggling with the modern times description of a dysfunctional brain. If this is the case, please read further. You'll be amazed to discover how common this problem is.

There are over 1 billion people around the world experiencing these various symptoms. The largest group is experiencing depression. Beyond that, mental health issues are impacting 15% of the world's children, 50% of the elderly, and will cause crippling effects to 25% of the global population over time.

Also, about a quarter of all adults have mental health issues. More than 1/6th of all people have an anxiety disorder, and about 1 in 10 adults has clinical depression. And, one in 10 adults, uses antidepressants. The money spent annually on antidepressants is over $2.5 billion dollars in the US. The cost of mental healthcare for depression alone is over 12.5% of all US healthcare spending.

Alzheimer's disease is estimated to impact about 1/3rd of all people over 80 years old, and will probably impact a higher number as people continue to suffer, and our modern world gets more toxic for them. The number has not reduced since first estimated.

Almost 10% of the children from age 8 into their mid-teens have been diagnosed with ADHD. Ten percent of all children now take Ritalin. Hopefully, this will reduce soon. Autism rates have increased from 1 in 3,333 in 1997 to more than 1 in 175 in the year 2000. Current statistics states that 1 in 88 children suffer from it. That is an amazing increase in 18 years. Learning disabilities now impact about 10% of all school-age children. The costs of managing these mental issues are amazingly high and put a financial drain on school districts' budgets.

Your Brain is NOT Broken, But Something is Wrong, Could it Be:
- Psychiatric disorders (emotional disturbance)?
- Neurological disorders (neurological impairment)?

Examples of what goes wrong:
- ADD
- ADHD
- Addictions
- Alzheimer's
- Anxiety
- Asperger's
- Autism

- Bipolar disease
- Dementia
- Depression
- Dyslexia
- Eating disorders
- Learning disabilities
- OCD - Obsessive-compulsive disorders
- Parkinson's
- Personality disorders

Pharmaceutical drugs for psychiatric or psychotropic reasons are the 2nd best-selling prescription drugs.

The first is cholesterol meds. Psychotropic drugs account for around 10% of the marketplace. Have our doctors become our drug dealers? The use of these drugs continues to grow as the big fix for whatever ails the mind.

The antidepressant class of drugs are the fastest growing of all prescribed drugs. In 2010, more than a quarter of a million prescriptions were filled for antidepressants. The Journal of the American Medical Association (JAMA) indicated that psychotropic medication use by outpatients increased significantly from 1985 to 1994, mostly from prescriptions written by psychiatrists. One drug, an antipsychotic called Abilify had sales of over $7 billion dollars. Pretty astounding for one drug. One article reported:

"There have been a number of changes in the prescription patterns of psychotropic medications among office-based physicians. Recent years have seen enormous changes in the health care system and in the availability and applications of new and older psychotropic drugs."

The Modern-Day Epidemic of Depression

It would be unique if no one you knew were depressed. It seems like everyone shows some signs of depression. It impacts and upsets the lives of 10% of all Americans, especially women. Approximate 4% of all Americans fit the statistics for severe depression, according to the CDC, and depression is the top cause of disability and suicide in the US. Suicide is the 10th top cause of death in the US, with over 100 people per day committing suicide. Suicide also has amazing costs in medical and work loss, exceeding $35 billion dollars. And, sadly only half of those diagnosed with depression get any form of treatment for it.

When people have depression, their quality of life suffers. Other mental health issues also impact life, but depression more so. In fact, depressed people suffer more than those with arthritis, lumbar back pain, diabetes, and so on. They lose all enjoyment of life's pleasures. They no longer enjoy things they used to enjoy. Losing the ability to appreciate family and friends, they are often overwhelmed trying to manage feelings and they respond with unprovoked anger or stuff their inner rage. They are sad and cry without any cause. Often, they have insomnia which makes the situation worse.

Medication is Not the Answer

Do we need a world filled with people who are living on stimulants, anti-depressants, anti-psychotics and medication to stimulate their memories? I don't think so. And, we certainly don't need everyone on Prozac. Still, these Big Pharma drugs are the main remedies known to psychiatric sciences at this point in time. Prescription medications help, no doubt about it, but it should only be reserved for when other less invasive therapies fail, like psychotherapy, nutrients and vitamins repletion, detoxification and the other WHYs are addressed.

Autism

Autism is growing in numbers. It could be the biggest social issue for parents in our generation. The statistics show there is a huge problem. The highest percentage of parents with autistic children is in high-tech firms in Silicon Valley ... Why?

We are not sure, but a leading researcher in autism, Dr. Robert Melillo, indicates that he believes it is related to neurological imbalances associated with both parents having left-brain (logic) dominance and very slow development of the right brain (creative) development. The theory indicates that unbalanced development of the two hemispheres of the brain is the probable cause.

This would explain the skills challenges that are symptomatic of autism. A child may be great at math but unable to draw. It also explains why autistic children are so withdrawn and have only minor socialization skills, and why autistic children are great at repetitive counting skills or movements, all which are left-brain functions.

Besides the parents being in science and technology in Silicon Valley, it is a place where scientists, programmers, engineers, from everywhere, meet. Other issues are that stress on pregnant working mothers, smoking, autoimmune diseases, fetal exposure to medications, toxic chemicals, and pesticides, plus vitamin deficiency, may be at cause. No one knows for certain.

However, what we do know is that American children are over medicated for mental conditions compared to other countries. Our rate of medication is 300% more than Germany, and 350% more than other European countries. If the medications were effective it would be an important plus – but realistically it leads to using other medications as adults, usually antidepressants.

Are Antidepressants the Worst Choice?

The majority of people who use antidepressants do not have a good response to use. Success with antidepressants is considered a 50% improvement in at least 50% of the symptoms. That's not the result that people would expect, and they do not even get that. More of them complain about the side effects of taking the medicine, than are happy with the result. Secondary effects include:

- fatigue
- loss of mental abilities
- increased risk of suicide
- insomnia
- nausea
- sexual dysfunction
- weight gain

The real question is, since we must ask one here, since depression is considered to be caused by a chemical imbalance in the brain is: *Why is there a chemical imbalance there at all?*

Psychiatry is not THE answer

Psychiatry believes that our life experiences or traumas control our moods and behaviors. However, the psychiatric disorders of our modern times are the results of chemical imbalances related to other organs and organ systems. These include the:

- immune system
- gastrointestinal tract
- endocrine system, and
- the ability of our liver to detoxify our body

No function of psychiatry, analysis, or therapy will eliminate depression resulting from:

- deficiencies in omega-3 fattyacid
- a lack of vitamin B12
- a low-functioning thyroid
- mercury toxicity

Modern psychiatry has become nothing more than a practice that attempts to alter the brain's chemistry using drugs, believing that mental illness can be summarized completely as brain chemistry imbalances, and they are dealing drug prescriptions for non-effective medications at high prices, trying to match drugs to the specific mental problem. It doesn't work like that.

Like most pharmaceutical medications, psychoactive ones are not problem solvers. They only suppress problems. If there is an imbalance in neurotransmission in the brain, there is a reason for that imbalance. Psychoactive medications do not solve these imbalances.

Let's see what's really behind this epidemic of chemical imbalances:
- Why do we have an epidemic of mentaldiseases?
- Are we defective in design?
- Can it be a lack of balance in our bodies?
- Are high-priced drugs a solution?

There must be some way to get to the causes, and balance our mental health, without medications that don't work anyway.

Functional Medicine Has a Solution

Functional Medicine believes the way to fix our brains lies, in the balance of health, in our bodies. The way to do that is to balance the issues impacting the health of our bodies – not using legal drugs to numb our brains.

Fix Your Body and You Will Fix Your Brain

Functional Medicine believes that the solution to the psychiatric and psychological problems lies in the improvement of the health and well-being of the body, not with psychoactive medications or psychotherapy. Brain disorders are nearly always due to systemic disorders in the body that impact the whole body including your brain.

The cure is not in the brain, but through the standards set up by Functional Medicine. The brain is impacted by hormonal imbalances (including thyroid issues, blood sugar issues) and detoxification issues, heavy metal exposure, gut problems, nutritional deficiencies, food sensitivities, lack of sleep, insufficient exercises, and too much stress. All of these can cause brain dysfunction – and all of these are the standard protocol of Functional Medicine. Each must be considered and treated for a long-lasting positive outcome.

When you repair the underlying bodily causes,
it allows the brain to heal, and brings
the neurotransmission system and brain
chemicals into balance.

When you realize that many of the psychiatric diseases are determined based on a list of symptoms without tests being performed, you also realize that psychiatry is the only medical field that does not require diagnostic blood tests or other bodily fluid tests to determine underlying cause. This is starting to change.

Functional medicine is the only concept that emphasizes that everything is connected. The brain is impacted by the organs and organ systems and vice-versa. Our stomach and intestines have now been connected to Alzheimer's, Parkinson's, and several other brain disorders. Studies show neurotransmitter production problems begin in the gut before impacting the brain. Again, toxicity, nutritional deficiency, blood sugar issues, and other dietary factors impact brain function, as well as lack of exercise, stress management, etc.

Functional Medicine is emerging as a modern treatment for mental and neurological issues, because the focus is on underlying causes rather than symptoms. It is a holistic approach involving assessment of imbalances throughout the patient's history, physical examinations, and the use of testing in a laboratory, as well as genetic factors. The environmental factors are also approached and a regimen of healthy diet, physical activities, meditation, nutrition, supplements and detoxification, among others, takes precedence for helping the patients regain physical, mental, and emotional balance.

No matter what the mental or neurological issue, whether it be depression, bipolar disorder, ADHD, ADD, Asperger's, Schizophrenia, Alzheimer's, Parkinson's, etc. therapies of Functional Medicine are effective at reducing symptoms and issues, without smoke and mirrors of psychoactive medications that have little positive effect and serious negative secondary effects.

Anxiety and depression and all other psychological problems benefit from Functional Medicine and Functional Nutrition. There is even an emerging specialty called Functional Psychiatry that incorporates all these precepts into their armamentarium.

If you have symptoms impacting your mental or physical health and want to get to the root cause, contact your nearest Functional Medicine practitioner. They are trained in helping you achieve the quality of life you desire and deserve.

METABOLIC SYNDROME
What is Metabolic Syndrome?

Metabolic syndrome is a group of symptoms including the existence of disorders that lead to CVD. It heightens the potential of acquiring diabetes, coronary disease, and having a stroke. Those with metabolic syndrome suffer issues with insulin uptake. The human body produces insulin to transport blood sugar to tissues while, simultaneously, using blood sugar's energy. Weight control issues are usually a problem for those suffering from metabolic syndrome, making it harder for tissues to utilize insulin. Metabolic syndrome is often a direct cause of diabetes.

Symptoms include:
- Adult females with a midsection bigger than 30 inches in circumference, or
- Adult males with a midsection bigger than 40 inches in circumference
- High blood pressure, over 130/85
- Elevated fasting blood sugar level at, or exceeding, 150
- High triglycerides greater than 199 mg/dl

HDL cholesterol (the "good" cholesterol), is believed to protect us against heart disease and can be raised through exercise, by eliminating smoking and through various dietary sources. HDL below 40 mg/dl for men and below 50 mg/dl for women is believed to increase the risk of having cardiovascular disease. Those who exercise regularly can have HDL values above 60 reducing their risk.

What Causes Metabolic Syndrome?

Many possible risk factors exist for metabolic syndrome; no one direct cause is known. They include:

- Obesity
- An inactive lifestyle
- Cholesterol issue and high triglycerides
- Hypertension,
- Insulin resistance

These components can effectively result in cardiovascular disease and Type II diabetes.

Different factors are considered to influence the development of metabolic syndrome including:

- Fats in the bloodstream
- Aging
- Abnormalities associated with levels of body fat
- Genetic influences

Factors associated with metabolic syndrome include:

- Aging. The chance of getting metabolic syndrome goes up with age.
- Ethnicity. African-Americans and Asian-Americans residing in the US have a higher tendency to developing metabolic syndrome. In addition, African-American women are usually 60% more at risk as compared to African-American men of the same age group.
- Body Mass Index (BMI) in excess of 30
- Genetics is often associated with diabetes.
- Smoking cigarettes
- Prolonged heavy drinking

- Unreleased stress and anxiety
- Post-menopausal situation
- Diets high in trans fats (especially partially hydrogenated oils)
- A sedentary lifestyle
- High blood pressure
- Cholesterol and Triglyceride issues
- Obesity

Exactly how is metabolic syndrome determined?

Standard evaluation includes:
- BMI (Body Mass Index)
- Elevated triglycerides
- Low HDL cholesterol
- High blood pressure (hypertension) or effects of antihypertensive medication
- Elevated fasting blood sugar
- Prothrombotic state (risk of blood clots)
- Insulin Resistance (inability of Insulin to work causing high blood sugar)
- Cholesterol particle sizes

Different diseases that could develop due to metabolic syndrome, other than Diabetes and Cardiovascular Disease include:
- Polycystic ovarian affliction
- Fatty liver disease
- Gallstones
- Asthma
- Sleeping disorder
- Melanomas

Conventional medicine treatment of Metabolic Syndrome:
- Eat a low fat and low salt diet
- Lose weight
- Exercise
- Medications to decrease blood pressure and blood sugar
- Quit smoking
- Low dose aspirin

Weight Loss Surgery

When other methods have failed, and one cannot lose weight with diet and exercise; and, medications have all failed, gastric bypass surgery is available for those with morbid obesity. One can likely normalize their weight, blood pressure, insulin uptake, lower their cholesterol, and get control of their triglycerides within about a year of having the surgery. It is, of course, the last resort if all of the most conservative of methods have failed.

Functional Medicine Approach

Fortunately, you are not doomed to be cut open. If you have metabolic syndrome and other problems are already showing: heart issues, pre-diabetes with high insulin or high blood sugar, cholesterol problems, etc. You can be treated in a different way, and have success reversing metabolic syndrome. We will cover diet and exercise, but there is more:

- Check your stomach, do you see a great deal of belly fat?
- Measure your hips, if you if your waist/hip ratio is unbalanced, then you have a problem. As a woman if your hips are over 37.5", and your abdomen is over 30", a problem exists. If you are a man if your hips are over

45" and your waste is over 40" - you have a problem.

- Start checking your insulin levels early in life. Especially if you are overweight, insulin levels increase many years before blood sugar or HbA1C become high. This is a pro-active way of preventing the development of Metabolic Syndrome and Diabetes.

Recommendations to resolve this includes:

- A healthy, low-glycemic diet
- A dietary change to a more plant-based diet
- A diet high in fiber
- A diet that is phytonutrient and omega-3 rich
- A diet with good quality protein like beans, nuts, seeds
- A diet with only lean animal protein (hopefully, organic and/or grass-fed)
- Completely ceasing cigarette smoking
- Severely restricting alcoholic consumption

Other things you must do:

- Exercise. (Check the exercise section in this book)
- Get a proper sleep, every night. The body heals itself during sleep; blood pressure normalizes during sleep. Your overall health improves through sleep
- Use supplements to improve sleep and create healthy cholesterol particle sizes. Include these:
- A multivitamin with enough Chromium, Biotin and Lipoic Acid
- 1000 mg of an omega-3 supplement, twice daily. 2000 IU of vitamin D3, twice daily
- 1200 mg of red yeast rice twice daily

- Broad-range, balanced concentration of plant sterols You will usually take 1 capsule with each meal
- 2-4 capsules of glucomannan 15 minutes before meals with a glass of water
- Consider using high-dose niacin or vitamin B3. This can only be done with a doctor's prescription
- Raise your HDL cholesterol, lower your LDL cholesterol and triglycerides, and work towards heightening particle size
- Use low-dose statins (cholesterol-reducing drugs if you suffer from heart disease or you are a man who has several risk factors. Be sure to monitor for damage to the muscle and liver.

For most people, this system is better than just using cholesterol medication. To lower your chance of heart disease you must address metabolic syndrome, and this can ONLY be done with a full diet and lifestyle change as outlined above.

Medication

Those with metabolic syndrome or who may be at risk might need medication at the beginning of their self-controlled program, and even later on if they have not had great success and not gotten good results with losing weight on their dietary program. This is especially so, if they are having trouble making their lifestyle changes, and they have not reduced their high blood pressure, reduced their cholesterol or triglyceride levels, and decreased their insulin resistance.

Medications that might be required include those to reduce blood pressure, heighten insulin metabolism, raise HDL cholesterol and lower LDL cholesterol, and to assist in losing weight.

CHRONIC RESPIRATORY CONDITIONS

Respiratory conditions impact our breathing. They impact the airways, and the lungs, and all the passages responsible for air movement in the body. The problems may be short-term in nature (acute) and cause illness, or last a long time (chronic), causing disabling effects, and death.

Common Chronic Respiratory Diseases

Chronic respiratory diseases are grouped in many different ways. One includes a rather large category of diseases that obstruct the air flow in and out of the lungs; these include:

- Asthma
- Bronchiectasis, (chronic or acute)
- Chronic obstructive pulmonary disease (COPD)
- Emphysema

Other respiratory issues can include:

- Chronic sinusitis
- Occupational lung disease
- And more

Asthma

Asthma is an inflammatory disease of the bronchi which is usually life-long. The symptoms are related to narrowing airways (bronchioconstriction), thickening of the walls of airways due to scarring, and increase of mucous in the respiratory system. It is a common illness and usually a severe chronic illness that puts patients and their families through considerable concern. Their symptoms cause them to limit their activity due to asthmatic attacks that often require trips to urgent or emergency care facilities. Asthma can be fatal.

Things get bad for those suffering asthma with viral infections, allergies to dust, outdoor pollens, dust mites, cockroaches, cigarette smoke, and even exercise. Some asthmatics react unfavorably to stressful conditions. Also, some pharmaceutical medications can trigger asthmatic reactions, i.e. beta-blockers, aspirin, and NSAIDs.

Further Causes of Asthma

It seems we are suffering from an epidemic of asthma, which affects such a huge range of people. Moreover, we wonder why. One reason might be that we've increased our Cesarean section births. More than 50% of newborns are delivered this way. When babies are not delivered vaginally, it appears that they do not get their mother's vaginal bacteria into their intestinal tract.

The vaginal bacteria seem to be important for the development of healthy, normal intestinal flora, and this is vital to developing a properly functioning immune system. In addition, infants in the US often do not get breast fed. That has been proven in Mexico, and other 3rd world countries to be an important factor in developing a newborn's healthy immune system. Formula is sometimes an allergen to newborns and they have to have a special formula that they are not allergic to.

Then, parents often give children breakfast cereal to snack on, after they finish their formula, and this contains gluten if served with milk, dairy – (Crunchy cereals are fed to babies who are teething in the US) and allergies develop, and later on Asthma.

These can cause an immune system problem in an infant. Then physicians often prescribe oral antibiotics for ear infections or sore throats which cause problems with developing normal, healthy intestinal flora. It continues to go on and on until allergies, inflammation, and further issues develop.

Research indicated that if pregnant women who had a genetic history of allergies were prescribed with acidophilus probiotics during the term of their pregnancy, there was a reduction of 50% in likelihood of their newborns developing allergies, asthma, a runny nose, and/or eczema. This is a simple approach which is low risk, low-cost, and effective.

Treatment of Asthma

Fortunately, asthma can be treated quite completely, and most sufferers end up achieving good control over it. When asthma is under control, patients are able to:

- Avoid symptoms during both day and night
- Use little to no medication
- Lead productive, active lives
- Enjoy normal or near-normal lung function
- Avoid serious flare-ups (attacks)

A stepwise approach takes into consideration the usefulness of available drugs, their risks, and their cost. Regular controller treatment, particularly with inhaled corticosteroid (ICS)-containing drugs, noticeably lessens the frequency and severity of asthma and the chance of attacks.

Asthma is a common ailment which affects all different levels of society. Athletes, leaders and celebrities, as well as normal people, lead successful, active lives with asthma.

COPD

Chronic Obstructive Pulmonary Disease causes a restriction in airflow within the lungs, and it often leads to a lack of breath, which isn't necessarily fixable even after treatment. COPD is usually a long-term illness that impacts many senior citizens.

Medical treatments for COPD include the following:

- Bronchodilators (beta2 agonists, Ipratropium bromide, and theophylline)
- Anti-Inflammatory Agents - Corticosteroids are often used to treat inflamed airways
- Mucolytics - guaifenesin, potassium iodide, and N-acetylcysteine.
- Antibiotics - used only for acute exacerbations.
- Oxygen - is the only treatment that has been shown to improve survival

Hay Fever

Hay fever is allergic rhinitis as a seasonal experience provoked by pollen. We have covered this in the section on allergies.

Bronchiectasis

Bronchiectasis (or Chronic Bronchiectasis) indicates an abnormal and permanent condition of the airways within the lungs. Those who are suffering from it often get infections as mucus collects in the lungs and the airways and stagnates.

There are some reasons it develops, including:
- COPD
- Cystic Fibrosis
- Low Antibody Levels
- Anesthesia- based pneumonia

Plus, infections such as:
- Tuberculosis
- Whooping Cough
- Measles

Treatment includes:

- Antibiotics
- Chest physiotherapy
- Bronchodilators
- Corticosteroid therapy,
- Expectorants and Mucus-Thinning Medicines
- Drinking plenty of fluid, especially water,
- Dietary supplementation,
- Oxygen
- Intravenous immunoglobulin or intravenous alpha1- antitrypsin (AAT) therapy
- Surgical therapies

Emphysema

Emphysema is a condition where the walls of air sacs in the lungs are damaged and continue to be damaged. The loss of tissue creates a collapse of small airways and permanently blocks the airflow, making it harder for the person to breathe. Emphysema, as well as chronic bronchitis, occurs in conjunction with chronic obstructive pulmonary disease (COPD).

What are the Signs and Symptoms?

The main sign of emphysema is a significant shortness of breath. This usually worsens as the disease progresses. Symptoms may also include:

- Chronic cough, usually occurs in the morning
- Lessened appetite and weight loss
- Lessened tolerance for physical activity
- Fatigue
- "Barrel Chest" appearance
- Abnormal breathing patterns

What are the causes of emphysema?

Emphysema happens when small air sacs in a person's lungs become damaged. Cigarette smoking is the most preventable and common cause of emphysema.

What is the conventional treatment?

- Stop smoking
- Avoid pollutants, lung irritants, and second-hand smoke
- Annual flu vaccination and vaccination for pneumonia (every five years)
- Bronchodilators
- Steroids.
- Antibiotics.
- Supplemental oxygen.

- Surgery
- Pulmonary rehabilitation

Chronic Sinusitis

Chronic sinusitis inflames the tissues lining one or more sinus cavities (within the bones of the face). This tends to occur when normal sinus draining is obstructed by swelling, excessive mucus, or possibly a deviated septum. It causes facial pain and is usually related to inflammation within the nose.

Treatments include:
- Saline nasal irrigation
- Nasal corticosteroids
- Oral or injected corticosteroids
- Decongestants.
- Over-the-counter pain relievers
- Aspirin desensitization
- Antibiotics
- Immunotherapy
- Surgery

Cystic Fibrosis

Cystic fibrosis (CF) is a genetic disorder where the mucous is very thick and sticky. This negatively impacts the lungs and other organs in the body. It is difficult to cleanse the mucous from the bronchial airways, and thus infections are involved, obstruction of breathing and problems that include brochiatesis and early death often result. Currently, the disease has no cure.

Treatments include:

- Antibiotics for treatment and prevention of lung infections
- Mucus-thinning medications to help cough up the phlegm, which increases the lung function
- Bronchodilators to keep airways open by relaxing muscles around the bronchial tubes
- Oral pancreatic enzymes to aid the digestive tract in absorption of nutrients
- Physical therapy for the chest
- Pulmonary rehabilitation
- Surgical and other procedures

Occupational Lung Diseases

Occupational lung diseases illnesses come from living and working in toxic environments including facilities with toxic dust or fumes, silica, asbestos, coal, and chemicals. This is normally a workplace disorder. Pneumoconiosis or lung scarring is usually caused by inhaling dust and is a very common form of occupational lung disease.

Treatment includes:
- Avoid any further exposure
- Corticosteroids
- Methotrexate
- Lung transplantation

Sleep Apnea

Sleep apnea is a respiratory condition impacting breathing while sleeping. Reduced airflow is one symptom that results in intermittent drops in oxygen levels in the blood causing the disorder. Patients with sleep apnea often don't know of their sleep-time breathing difficulties. When asthmatics has sleep apnea, they can die in their sleep without symptoms.

Treatment:
- Continuous positive airway pressure (CPAP)
- Expiratory positive airway pressure (EPAP)
- Adjustable airway pressure devices
- Oral appliances
- Surgery - Tissue removal
- Surgery - Jaw repositioning
- Surgery - Implants
- Surgery - Fabricating a new airway (tracheotomy)

Pulmonary Fibrosis

Pulmonary fibrosis is lung scarring and tissue thickening. It impacts oxygen transfer into the bloodstream. Often the cause is unknown. When this scarring occurs, it is called idiopathic pulmonary fibrosis.

Treatments:
- Antihistamines
- Decongestants
- Non-narcotic analgesics like aspirin
- NSAIDs
- Nasal sprays – but there is a rebound effect of increased congestion
- Steroidal nasal sprays

Functional Medicine for Respiratory Disorders

Addressing the Root Causes of Asthma

I have been able to help many patients improve their asthma symptoms by addressing these underlying and root causes. The questions are, "what causes asthma and what can be done about it? How can we eliminate these symptoms?"

Asthma is a huge issue today. It impacts 8 ½% of the population, or more than 25 million Americans and it is growing every day in the US. This growth is because of heightened environmental poisons, growing pollution, growth in food sensitivities and gut issues, food dyes and other additives, heightened use of antibiotics and medications, and growing use of foods with changed proteins and other weird ingredients. All these factors can and do lead to or exacerbate asthma.

So, what can be done to combat the rise of respiratory diseases? Functional Medicine is a scientific-based method because it focuses on finding root causes, instead of suppressing symptoms like allopathic medicine that's based on pharmaceutical and surgical treatments. The simple concept of Functional Medicine – if you are stepping on a thumbtack, don't take a pain pill – remove it and you do not need the medication. This is a simple theory, missed by so many physicians. Functional Medicine - fixes the cause.

How to Cure Your Respiratory Disease

Eliminate the bad stuff in life that could be possible causes, we've mentioned just about all of them here in this segment on Respiratory Diseases. Also, put things in your body that it needs to heal, clean up your digestive system. If there are yeast issues, take probiotics after cleaning your gut out.

Asthma is one of the easier things to eliminate in your life; others are more difficult. However, go see your Functional Medicine doctor, discover the cause of your disease, rebalance your body, let your immune system rebuild – it has been working overtime fighting for your life. Chill – and let the natural methodology of Functional Medicine work positively for you.

RECOMMENDED READING

- The Blood Sugar Solution: The UltraHealthy Program for Losing Weight, Preventing Disease, and Feeling Great Now!
Hardcover – Large Print, February 28, 2012
by Mark Hyman
Publisher: Little, Brown and Company; Reprint edition (December 30, 2014)
ISBN-10: 0316196177
ISBN-13: 978-0316196178

- Grain Brain: The Surprising Truth about Wheat, Carbs, and Sugar--Your Brain's Silent Killers Hardcover – September 17, 2013
by David Perlmutter (Author), Kristin Loberg (Contributor)
Publisher: Little, Brown and Company; 1 edition (September 17, 2013)
ISBN-10: 031623480X
ISBN-13: 978-0316234801

- Wheat Belly: Lose the Wheat, Lose the Weight, and Find Your Path Back to Health Hardcover – August 30, 2011
by William Davis
Publisher: Rodale Books; 1 edition (August 30, 2011)
ISBN-10: 1609611543
ISBN-13: 978-1609611545

- The Autoimmune Solution: Prevent and Reverse the Full Spectrum of Inflammatory Symptoms and Diseases Hardcover
  – January 27, 2015
  by Amy Myers (Author)
  Publisher: HarperOne; 1 edition (January 27, 2015)
  Language: English
  ISBN-10: 0062347470
  ISBN-13: 978-0062347473

- The Great Cholesterol Myth: Why Lowering Your Cholesterol Won't Prevent Heart Disease-and the Statin-Free Plan That Will Paperback – November 1, 2012
  by Jonny Bowden (Author), Stephen Sinatra (Author)
  Publisher: Fair Winds Press; 1 edition (November 1, 2012)
  Language: English
  ISBN-10: 1592335217
  ISBN-13: 978-1592335213

- Clinical Nutrition: A Functional Approach Paperback – 2004 by Dan Lukaczer (Author)
  Publisher: IFM; 2nd Edition edition (2004)
  ISBN-10: 0977371328
  ISBN-13: 978-0977371327

- Supplement Your Prescription: What Your Doctor Doesn't Know About Nutrition Paperback – October 15, 2007
  by Hyla Cass (Author)
  Publisher: Basic Health Publications; 1st edition (October 15, 2007)
  ISBN-10: 1591202272
  ISBN-13: 978-1591202271

- What You Must Know About Vitamins, Minerals, Herbs & More: Choosing the Nutrients That Are Right for You Paperback – September 15, 2007
  by M.D. Pamela Wartian Smith (Author)
  Publisher: Square One Publishers; 1 edition (September 15, 2007)
  ISBN-10: 0757002331
  ISBN-13: 978-0757002335

- Textbook of Functional Medicine Hardcover – 2005 by Sidney MacDonald Baker (Author), Peter Bennett (Author), Jeffrey S. Bland (Author), Leo Galland (Author), Robert J. Hedaya (Author), Mark Houston (Author), Mark Hyman (Author), Jay Lombard (Author), Robert Rountree (Author), Alex Vasquez (Author) Publisher: Institute for Functional Medicine; 2nd edition (2005)
  ISBN-10: 0977371301
  ISBN-13: 978-0977371303

- BEYOND FOODS: The Handbook of Functional Nutrition Kindle Edition
  by Barbara Swanson (Author)
  Publisher: Original Skin Organics; 1 edition (June 15, 2014)
  Publication Date: June 15, 2014
  Sold by: Amazon Digital Services, Inc.
  ASIN: B00L1M0GZ0

- Enzymes & Enzyme Therapy: How to Jump-Start Your Way to Lifelong Good Health by Anthony Cichoke (Author), Abram Hoffer MD (Author), Anthony J. Cichoke DC (Author)
  Publisher: McGraw-Hill Education; 2 edition (April 22, 2000)
  ISBN-10: 0658002902
  ISBN-13: 978-0658002908

- Eat Light & Feel Bright: Microalgae Solutions for
Individual and Planetary Health by Jeffrey Bruno, PhD.
Publisher: Pacific Psychological Care (February 12, 2014)
ISBN-10: 0991392507
ISBN-13: 978-0991392506

- Mycelium Running: How Mushrooms Can Help Save
the World by Paul Stamets (Author)
Publisher: Ten Speed Press; First edition (October 1, 2005)
ISBN-10: 1580085792
ISBN-13: 978-1580085793

- Food Energetics: The Spiritual, Emotional, and
Nutritional Power of What We Eat. By Steve Gagné
(Author)
Publisher: Healing Arts Press; 3 edition
ISBN-10: 1594772428
ISBN-13: 978-1594772429

- Salt Your Way to Health, 2nd Edition Paperback use
pre-formatted date that complies with legal
requirement from media matrix – 2006
by David Brownstein, M.D.
Publisher: Medical Alternative Press; 2 edition (2006)
ISBN-13: 978-0966088243
ASIN: B000R8ZTGK

- The Yeast Syndrome: How to Help Your Doctor Identify &
Treat the Real Cause of Your Yeast-Related Illness Mass
Market Paperback use pre-formatted date that complies
with legal requirement from media matrix – Oct. 1, 1986
by John P. Trowbridge (Author), Morton Walker (Author)
Publisher: Bantam (October 1, 1986)
ISBN-10: 0553277510
ISBN-13: 978-0553277517

REFERENCES

Introduction

Bergland, C. (2013). *Mindfulness Made Simple.* [online] Psychology Today. Available at: https://www.psychologytoday.com/blog/the-athletes-way/201303/mindfulness-made-simple [Accessed 2 Aug. 2015].

Chapter 1

Barlow, S. (2012). *Understanding the Healer Archetype : Susanna Barlow.* [online] Susannabarlow.com. Available at: http://susannabarlow.com/on-archetypes/ understanding-the-healer-archetype/ [Accessed 3 Aug. 2015].

Dashú, M. (2006). *Woman Shaman.* [online] Suppressedhistories.net. Available at: http:// www.suppressedhistories.net/articles/womanshaman.html [Accessed 3 Aug. 2015].

Lambert, T. (2014). *A Brief History of Medicine.* [online] Localhistories.org. Available at: http://www.localhistories.org/medicine.html [Accessed 3 Aug. 2015].

Bamber, G. (2001). *HistoryWorld - History and Timelines.* [online] Historyworld.net. Available at: http://www.historyworld.net/ [Accessed 3 Aug. 2015].

Woolcott, V. (2015). *History Of Shamanism | Shamanic Journey.* [online] Shamanicjourney.com. Available at: http://www.shamanicjourney.com/history-of-shamanism [Accessed 3 Aug. 2015].

Healthandhealingny.org, (n.d.). *Ayurveda - History and Philosophy.* [online] Available at: http://www.healthandhealingny.org/tradition_healing/ayurveda-history.html [Accessed 3 Aug. 2015].

Chapter 2

Aafa-md.org, (2015). *Allergy Basics:: Asthma & Allergy Foundation of America of Maryland - Greater Washington DC.* [online] Available at: http://www.aafa-md.org/allergy_basics.htm [Accessed 3 Aug. 2015].

AIHM, (2015). *Academy of Integrative Health & Medicine: Faculty Bios.* [online] Available at: http://aihm.org/education/faculty-bios/ [Accessed 3 Aug. 2015].

Aldokkan.com, (2015). *Egyptian Herbs and Remedies.* [online] Available at: http://www. aldokkan.com/science/herbal_remedies.htm [Accessed 3 Aug. 2015].

Anon, (n.d.). [online] Available at: http://www.brandyaugustine.com/journal/2014/7/7/3- ways-dietary-fiber-helps-maintainhormone-balance [Accessed 3 Aug. 2015].

Anon, (n.d.). [online] Available at: http://www.chemicalbodyburden.org/whatisbb.htm [Accessed 3 Aug. 2015].

Anon, (n.d.). [online] Available at: http://www.patheos.com/blogs/faithonthecouch/2014/05/ faith-spirituality-belief-religionwhats-the-difference/ [Accessed 3 Aug. 2015]

Anon, (n.d.). [online] Available at: https://elissagoodman.com/lifestyle/how-to-stop- attacking-yourself-nine-steps-to-healautoimmune-disease/ [Accessed 3 Aug. 2015].

Anon, (n.d.). [online] Available at: http://theunboundedspirit.com/how-to-stop-attacking- yourself-9-steps-to-healautoimmune-disease/ [Accessed 3 Aug. 2015].

Anon, (n.d.). [online] Available at: http://drliesa.com/medical-services/allergy-testing-and- relief/ [Accessed 3 Aug. 2015].

Anon, (n.d.). [online] Available at: http://drhyman.com/blog/2011/01/28/seven-tips-to-fix- your-cholesterol-withoutmedication/#close [Accessed 3 Aug. 2015

Chapter 3

Antiageingconference.com, (n.d.). *Anti-Aging Conference - Preventative Health Care.* [online] Available at:
http://www.antiageingconference.com/index.html?pg=braverman [Accessed 3 Aug. 2015].

Businessweek.com, (n.d.). *List of Private Companies Worldwide, Letter - Businessweek.* [online] Available at:
http://www.bloomberg.com/research/common/symbollookup/ symbollookup.asp?lookuptype=private&region=all [Accessed 3 Aug. 2015].

Cdc.gov, (n.d.). *CDC - DHDSP - Heart Disease Facts.* [online] Available at:
http://www.cdc.gov/ heartdisease/facts.htm [Accessed 3 Aug. 2015].

Cfhll.com, (n.d.). *Welcome to The Center For Healthy Living and Longevity :..* [online] Available at: http://www.cfhll.com/bio_p_smith.html [Accessed 3 Aug. 2015].

Dillon, J. (n.d.). *From the potion to the pill > Features > Spring 2007 | Yale Medicine.* [online] Yalemedicine.yale.edu. Available at:
http://yalemedicine.yale.edu/spring2007/features/ feature/51660/ [Accessed 3 Aug. 2015].

Gilhooly, C., Das, S., Golden, J., McCrory, M., Dallal, G., Saltzman, E., Kramer, F. and Roberts, S. (2007). Food cravings and energy regulation: the characteristics of craved foods and their relationship with eating behaviors and weight change during 6 months of dietary energy restriction. *Int J Obes Relat Metab Disord,* 31(12), pp.1849-1858.

Ginasthma.org, (n.d.). *Pocket Guide for Asthma Management and Prevention | Documents / Resources | GINA.* [online] Available at:
http://www.ginasthma.org/documents/1/ Pocket-Guide-for-Asthma-Management-andPrevention [Accessed 3 Aug. 2015].

GSK, (n.d.). [online] Available at: http://www.gsk.com/about/history.htm [Accessed 3 Aug. 2015].

http://en.wikipedia.orgHealthy.net, (2015). *Biography: Leo Galland MD, FACN.* [online] Available at:
http://www.healthy.net/Author_Biography/Leo_Galland_MD_FACN/125 [Accessed 3 Aug. 2015].

Herne, (n.d.). *Herbal History at The Celtic Connection.* [online] Wicca.com. Available at:
http://wicca.com/celtic/herbal/history.htm [Accessed 3 Aug. 2015].

Hsph.harvard.edu, (n.d.). *Fats and Cholesterol | The Nutrition Source | Harvard T.H. Chan School of Public Health.* [online] Available at: http://www.hsph.harvard.edu/ nutritionsource/fats-and-cholesterol-1/ [Accessed 3 Aug. 2015].

Jenn Mears, N., Wachter, H., Dregni, M., Cox, C. and Millard, E. (2013). *Functional-Medicine Roundup.* [online] Experience Life. Available at: https://experiencelife.com/functional- medicine-round-up/ [Accessed 3 Aug. 2015].

KGaA, M. (n.d.). *History - EMD Group.* [online] Merckgroup.com. Available at: http://www. merckgroup.com/en/company/history/history.html [Accessed 3 Aug. 2015].

Lactose Intolerance. (n.d.). [online] Available at: http://www.bpac.org.nz/BPJ/2007/October/ docs/bpj9_lactose_pages_30-35.pdf [Accessed 3 Aug. 2015].

Lmreview.com, (n.d.). *Articles | Longevity and Aging Research Articles | Longevity Medicine Review.* [online] Available at: http://www.lmreview.com/articles/ [Accessed 3 Aug. 2015].

Mark Hyman, M., Labatt, G., David Perlmutter, M., Trespicio, T., Weintraub, P., Jenn Mears, N., Wachter, H., Dregni, M. and Cox, C. (2008). *Functional Wellness, Part 5: The Body- Mind Connection.* [online] Experience Life. Available at: https://experiencelife.com/ article/functional-wellness-part-5-the-body-mind-connection/ [Accessed 3 Aug. 2015].

MedicineNet, (2012). Toxicity. [online] Available at: http://www.medicinenet.com/script/ main/art.asp?articlekey=34093 [Accessed 3 Aug. 2015].

MindBodyGreen, (2013). *10 Signs You Have An Autoimmune Disease + How To Reverse It.* [online] Available at: http://www.mindbodygreen.com/0-8843/10-signs-you-have-an- autoimmune-disease-how-to-reverse-it.html [Accessed 3 Aug. 2015].

MindBodyGreen, (2013). *10 Signs You Have An Autoimmune Disease + How To Reverse It.* [online] Available at: http://www.mindbodygreen.com/0-8843/10-signs-you-have-an- autoimmune-disease-how-to-reverse-it.html [Accessed 3 Aug. 2015].

Pauling, L. (n.d.). *About Linus Pauling.* [online] Hearttechnology.com. Available at: http:// www.hearttechnology.com/pauling_scientific_achievements.html [Accessed 3 Aug. 2015].

Scientific American - Science News, Articles, and Information, (2015). *Science News, Articles, and Information - Scientific American.* [online] Available at: http://www.scientificamerican.com/article.cfm?id [Accessed 3 Aug. 2015].

smart-publications.com, (n.d.). [online] Available at: http://www.smart-publications.com/ articles/dr-bruce-ames-proves-his-triage-theory-ofmicronutrients-with-vitamin [Accessed 3 Aug. 2015].

Stone, K. (n.d.). *All About Viibryd.* [online] About.com Money. Available at: http://pharma. about.com/od/FDA/a/All-About-Viibryd.htm [Accessed 3 Aug. 2015].

Walston, J. (n.d.). *Functional Medicine and Cancer.* [online] Jeannine Walston. Available at: http://jeanninewalston.com/integrative-cancer-care/body/integrative-cancer-medicine- systems/functional-medicine-and-cancer/ [Accessed 3 Aug. 2015].

Wikipedia, (2015). *Main Page.* [online] Available at: https://en.wikipedia.org/wiki/Main_ Page [Accessed 3 Aug. 2015].

Ashlandmd.com, (2015). *Ashland's Comprehensive Family Medicine:: David Scott Jones.* [online] Available at: http://www.ashlandmd.com/DavidScottJones [Accessed 3 Aug. 2015].

Benjamin Wedro, F. (2015). *Gastroenteritis (Stomach Flu): Is it Contagious?* [online] eMedicineHealth. Available at: http://www.emedicinehealth.com/gastroenteritis/article_ em.htm [Accessed 3 Aug. 2015].

Botha, L. (2015). *Hormone Imbalance- The Silent Epidemic | BellaSpark.* [online] Bellaspark.com. Available at: http://bellaspark.com/articles/entry/hormone-imbalance-the-silent-epidemic/ [Accessed 3 Aug. 2015].

Chapter 4
Conger, C. (2015). *How Food Cravings Work.* [online] HowStuffWorks. Available at: http:// science.howstuffworks.com/innovation/edible-innovations/food-craving.htm [Accessed 3 Aug. 2015].
David Perlmutter M.D., (2015). *The Expert on Brain Health Talks Gluten Intolerance & Allergies.* [online] Available at: http://www.drperlmutter.com/about/bio/ [Accessed 3 Aug. 2015].
Emmons, E. (2015). *Bronchiectasis Treatment & Management: Approach Considerations, Supportive Treatment, Antibiotic Therapy.* [online] Emedicine.medscape.com. Available at: http://emedicine.medscape.com/article/296961-treatment [Accessed 3 Aug. 2015].
Emmons, E. (2015). *Medical Treatment for COPD - Chronic Obstructive Pulmonary Disease (COPD) - HealthCommunities.com.* [online] Healthcommunities.com. Available at: http://www.healthcommunities.com/copd/medical-treatment.shtml [Accessed 3 Aug. 2015].
Eufic.org, (2015). *Dietary fibre – what's its role in a healthy diet? (EUFIC).* [online] Available at: http://www.eufic.org/article/en/nutrition/fibre/artid/dietary-fibre-role-healthy-diet/ [Accessed 3 Aug. 2015].
Functionalmedicine.org, (2015). *Institute for Functional Medicine > What is Functional Medicine?* [online] Available at: https://www.functionalmedicine.org/about/whatisfm/ [Accessed 3 Aug. 2015].
Functionalmedicine.org, (2015). *Institute for Functional Medicine > Jeffrey Bland, PhD.* [online] Available at: https://www.functionalmedicine.org/AboutFM/ourteam/faculty/ bios/bland/ [Accessed 3 Aug. 2015].
Functionalmedicine.org, (2015). *Institute for Functional Medicine > Mark Hyman, MD.* [online] Available at: https://www.functionalmedicine.org/AboutFM/ourteam/faculty/ bios/hyman/ [Accessed 3 Aug. 2015].
Functionalmedicine.org, (2015). *Institute for Functional Medicine > Bethany Hays, MD.* [online] Available at: https://www.functionalmedicine.org/AboutFM/ourteam/faculty/ bios/Hays/ [Accessed 3 Aug. 2015].

Functionalmedicine.org, (2015). *Institute for Functional Medicine > Functional Medicine and Integrative Medicine.* [online] Available at: https://www.functionalmedicine.org/page. aspx?id=781 [Accessed 3 Aug. 2015].

Functionalmedicine.org, (2015). *Institute for Functional Medicine > Working with a Functional Medicine Practitioner.* [online] Available at: https://www.functionalmedicine. org/about/working_with_a_functional/ [Accessed 3 Aug. 2015].

Functionalmedicine.org, (2015). *Institute for Functional Medicine > What is Functional Medicine?* [online] Available at: https://www.functionalmedicine.org/about/whatisfm/ [Accessed 3 Aug. 2015].

Grisanti, R. (2015). *Leaky Gut: Can This Be Destroying Your Health?* [online] Functionalmedicineuniversity.com. Available at: http://www.functionalmedicineuniversity.com/ public/Leaky-Gut.cfm [Accessed 3 Aug. 2015].

Hak E, e. (2015). *Association of childhood attention-deficit/hyperactivity disorder with atopic diseases and skin infections? A matched case-control study using the ... - PubMed - NCBI.* [online] Ncbi.nlm.nih.gov. Available at: http://www.ncbi.nlm.nih.gov/ pubmed/23886227 [Accessed 3 Aug. 2015].

Holistichealthbayarea.com, (2015). *Metabolic Syndrome Treatment With Nutrition and Functional Medicine | Functional Medicine Bay Area - Holistic Health Bay Area (650) 394- 7470 - San Carlos CA 94070.* [online] Available at: http://www.holistichealthbayarea.com/ blog/metabolic-syndrome-treatment/ [Accessed 3 Aug. 2015].

Hsph.harvard.edu, (2015). *Fats and Cholesterol | The Nutrition Source | Harvard T.H. Chan School of Public Health.* [online] Available at: http://www.hsph.harvard.edu/ nutritionsource/fats-and-cholesterol-1/ [Accessed 3 Aug. 2015].

Julie Warren, P. (2015). *Does Exercise Release a Chemical in the Brain?* [online] LIVESTRONG.COM. Available at: http://www.livestrong.com/article/320144-does- exercise-release-a-chemical-in-the-brain/ [Accessed 3 Aug. 2015].

Kotsanis Institute, (2015). *Kotsanis Institute.* [online] Available at: http://www. kotsanisinstitute.com/services/hormone-imbalances [Accessed 3 Aug. 2015].

Life Extension.org, (2015). *Inflammation (Chronic).* [online] Available at: https://www.lef. org/protocols/health-concerns/chronic-inflammation/Page-01 [Accessed 3 Aug. 2015].

LifeExtension.com, (2015). *Highest Quality Vitamins And Supplements - Life Extension.* [online] Available at: http://www.lifeextension.com/ [Accessed 3 Aug. 2015].

Main Differences Between IgE and IgG Allergies. (2015). [online] Available at: http://www. greatplainslaboratory.com/home/eng/e-newsletter/igg_vs_ige.pdf [Accessed 3 Aug. 2015].

Mayoclinic.org, (2015). *Mayo Clinic.* [online] Available at: http://www.mayoclinic.org/ [Accessed 3 Aug. 2015].

Monell.org, (2015). *Monell Chemical Senses Center.* [online] Available at: http://www.monell.org/ researchoverview_h.htm [Accessed 3 Aug. 2015].

Naturalhealthcareanddiagnostics.com, (2015). *Functional Medicine Approach to Autoimmune Diseases (lupus, arthritis).* [online] Available at: http://naturalhealthcareanddiagnostics.com/ thyroid-problems/approach-to-autoimmune-diseases/ [Accessed 3 Aug. 2015].

Nhs.uk, (2015). *Benefits of exercise - Live Well - NHS Choices.* [online] Available at: http:// www.nhs.uk/Livewell/fitness/Pages/Whybeactive.aspx [Accessed 3 Aug. 2015].

Patient, (2015). *Physical Activity For Health. Exercise advice information | Patient.* [online] Available at: http://patient.info/health/physical-activity-for-health [Accessed 3 Aug. 2015].

Pfizer.com, (2015). *History | Pfizer: One of the world's premier biopharmaceutical companies.* [online] Available at: http://www.pfizer.com/about/history/history [Accessed 3 Aug. 2015].

Pharmacy.wsu.edu, (2015). *Home | WSU College of Pharmacy.* [online] Available at: http://www.pharmacy.wsu.edu/ [Accessed 3 Aug. 2015].

Psychologytoday.com, (2015). *Psychology Today: Health, Help, Happiness + Find a Therapist.* [online] Available at: https://www.psychologytoday.com/ [Accessed 3 Aug. 2015].

RnA Superfood, (2015). *Obsolescing Supplements, One Drop at a Time - RnA Drops Testimonial Review.* [video] Available at: http://www.viewtubetrain.com/watch.php?v=148009 [Accessed 3 Aug. 2015].

Roddick, J. (2015). *Autoimmune Disease.* [online] Healthline. Available at: http://www. healthline.com/health/autoimmune-disorders?toptoctest=expand#Overview1 [Accessed 3 Aug. 2015].

Science.jrank.org, (2015). *Respiratory Diseases - Treatments.* [online] Available at: http://science.jrank.org/pages/5832/Respiratory-Diseases-Treatments.html [Accessed 3 Aug. 2015].

Smith, A. (2015). *What Are the Normal Levels of LDL & HDL? | eHow.* [online] eHow. Available at: http://www.ehow.com/about_5089633_normal-levels-ldl-hdl.html [Accessed 3 Aug. 2015].

Stress.org, (2015). *What is stress? | The American Institute of Stress.* [online] Available at: http://www.stress.org/what-is-stress/ [Accessed 3 Aug. 2015].

The Physicians Committee, (2015). *| The Physicians Committee.* [online] Available at: http://www.pcrm.org/health/cancer-resources/diet-cancer/nutrition/how-fiber-helps- protectagainst-cancer [Accessed 3 Aug. 2015].

Thestar.com.my, (2015). *Malaysia Business & Finance News, Stock Updates | The Star Online.* [online] Available at: http://www.thestar.com.my/Business/ [Accessed 3 Aug. 2015].

Yourmedicaldetective.com, (2015). *What is Functional Medicine?* [online] Available at: http://www.yourmedicaldetective.com/public/department50.cfm [Accessed 3 Aug. 2015].

Baker, S. (2014). *Sydney M. Baker, M.D.From Yale Medical School to author, to public speaker and a very special focus on children.* [online] Betterhealthusa.com. Available at: http://www.betterhealthusa.com/public/226.cfm [Accessed 3 Aug. 2015].

Hardin, J. (2014). *Allergies & Your Gut - Good gut health is central to our overall well-being.* [online] Allergies & Your Gut. Available at: http://allergiesandyourgut.com/ [Accessed 3 Aug. 2015].

Mayoclinic.org, (2014). *Meditation: Take a stress-reduction break wherever you are - Mayo Clinic.* [online] Available at: http://www.mayoclinic.org/tests-procedures/meditation/ in-depth/meditation/art-20045858 [Accessed 3 Aug. 2015].

Stephen Sinatra, F. (2014). *Dr. Stephen Sinatra's Informational Site - Heart MD Institute.* [online] Heartmdinstitute.com. Available at: http://www.heartmdinstitute.com/about- us/stephen-sinatra-md-facc [Accessed 3 Aug. 2015].

Who.int, (2014). *WHO | Dioxins and their effects on human health.* [online] Available at: http://www.who.int/mediacentre/factsheets/fs225/en/ [Accessed 3 Aug. 2015].

Blum, S. (2013). *Functional Medicine for Autoimmune Diseases.* [online] Utne. Available at: http://www.utne.com/mind-and-body/autoimmune-diseases-ze0z1309zcalt. aspx?PageId=4 [Accessed 3 Aug. 2015].

Colosimo, J. (2013). *Nutrition and Chronic Inflammation | Invision Health Functional Medicine.* [online] Invision Health. Available at: http://www.invisionhealth.com/ nutrition-chronic-disease-inflammation/ [Accessed 3 Aug. 2015].

Colosimo, J. (2013). *Nutrition and Chronic Inflammation | Invision Health Functional Medicine.* [online] Invision Health. Available at: http://www.invisionhealth.com/ nutrition-chronic-disease-inflammation/ [Accessed 3 Aug. 2015].

Gabriel, G. (2013). *Hans Selye: The Discovery of Stress - Brain Connection.* [online] Brain Connection. Available at: http://brainconnection.brainhq.com/2013/04/05/hans-selye- the-discovery-of-stress/ [Accessed 3 Aug. 2015].

Hill, D. (2013). *Functional Medicine Starts with Good Detoxification - Paleo Lifestyle DoctorPaleo Lifestyle Doctor.* [online] Paleolifestyledoctor.com. Available at: http:// paleolifestyledoctor.com/functional-medicine-starts-good-detoxification/ [Accessed 3 Aug. 2015].

Jacobs, (2013). *Increased Lipolysis Fat Oxidation & Weight Loss | LIVESTRONG.COM.* [online] LIVESTRONG.COM. Available at: http://www.livestrong.com/article/201038- increased-lipolysis-fat-oxidation-weight-loss/ [Accessed 3 Aug. 2015].

Mark Hyman, M. (2013). *Breathe Easy — Addressing the Root Causes of Asthma.* [online] Dr. Mark Hyman. Available at: http://drhyman.com/blog/2013/09/17/breathe-easy- addressing-root-causes-asthma/ [Accessed 3 Aug. 2015].

McClure, B. (2013). *::: Cloquet Natural Foods and Wellness Center Blog :::.* [online] Cloquetwellness.blogspot.ca. Available at: http://cloquetwellness.blogspot.ca/ [Accessed 3 Aug. 2015].

Sayin, I., Cingi, C., Oghan, F., Baykal, B. and Ulusoy, S. (2013). Complementary Therapies in Allergic Rhinitis. *ISRN Allergy,* 2013, pp.1-9.

Dinarello, C. (2011). A clinical perspective of IL-1β as the gatekeeper of inflammation. *European Journal of Immunology,* 41(5), pp.1203-1217.

Chapter 5

Lad, V. (2012). *Ayurvedic perspectives on selected pathologies.* Albuquerque, NM: Ayurvedic Press. Medicine, R. (2012). *Brain Health.* [online] San Jose Functional Medicine. Available at:

> http://sanjosefuncmed.com/brain-health/ [Accessed 3 Aug. 2015].

Copingmag.com, (2011). *Coping with Allergies & Asthma - Print Article.* [online] Available at:

> http://copingmag.com/ana/index.php/site/print_article/www.AllergyAndAsthmaRe lie [Accessed 3 Aug. 2015].

Davis, W. (2011). *Wheat belly.* Emmaus, Penn.: Rodale.

Mama, K. (2011). *Interview with Wheat Belly Author Dr. William Davis.* [online] Wellness Mama. Available at. http://wellnessmama.com/3486/dr-william-davis-wheat-belly/ [Accessed 3 Aug. 2015].

Tschopp, J. (2011). Mitochondria: Sovereign of inflammation? *European Journal of Immunology,* 41(5), pp.1196-1202.

Windgassen et al, (2011). *Inflammation (Chronic) - Mitochondrial Dysfunction , Enzymes, Eicosanoids - Life Extension Health Concern.* [online] LifeExtension.com. Available at: http://www.lifeextension.com/Protocols/Health-Concerns/Chronic-Inflammation/ Page-01 [Accessed 3 Aug. 2015].

Mark Hyman, M. (2010). *Is There Toxic Waste In Your Body? - Dr. Mark Hyman.* [online] Dr. Mark Hyman. Available at: http://drhyman.com/blog/2010/05/19/is-there-toxic- waste-in-your-body-2/ [Accessed 3 Aug. 2015].

Survivingcipro.com, (2010). *Your Survival Stories | Surviving Cipro.* [online] Available at: http://www.survivingcipro.com/useful-information/staying-positive/your-success- stories/ [Accessed 3 Aug. 2015].

Walsh, R. (2010). *A history of: The pharmaceutical industry.* [online] pharmaphorum. Available at: http://www.pharmaphorum.com/articles/a-history-of-the-pharmaceutical- industry [Accessed 3 Aug. 2015].

Caruso, D. (2009). *Mark Hyman, MD: Healing the Broken Brain Syndrome - Life Extension.* [online] LifeExtension.com. Available at: http://www.lef.org/magazine/2009/3/mark- hyman-healing-broken-brain-syndrome/page-01 [Accessed 3 Aug. 2015].

Prasher, S. (2009). *Canada Loses Medical Icon Dr. Abram Hoffer | Orthomolecular Health.* [online] Orthomolecularhealth.com. Available at: https://www.orthomolecularhealth. com/canada-loses-medical-icon-dr-abram-hoffer/ [Accessed 3 Aug. 2015].

Lad, V. and Durve, A. (2008). *Marma points of Ayurveda.* Albuquerque, N.M.: Ayurvedic Press.

Mills, H., Reiss, N. And Dombeck, P, M. (2008). *Meditation for Stress Reduction - Dealing with Stress and Anxiety Management ?EUR" Coping Mechanisms from MentalHelp.net.* [online] Mentalhelp.net. Available at: https://www.mentalhelp.net/articles/meditation- for-stress-reduction/ [Accessed 3 Aug. 2015].

Maintz, L. and Novak, N. (2007). *Histamine and histamine intolerance. The American Journal of Clinical Nutrition,* [online] 85(5), pp.1185-1196. Available at: http://ajcn.nutrition. org/content/85/5/1185.long [Accessed 3 Aug. 2015].

Eufic.org, (2006). *Food allergy and food intolerance (EUFIC).* [online] Available at: http:// www.eufic.org/article/en/expid/basics-food-allergy-intolerance/ [Accessed 3 Aug. 2015].

Squires, S. (2006). *Sally Squires - Give In, but Not Completely.* [online] Washingtonpost.com.
Available at: http://www.washingtonpost.com/wp-dyn/content/article/2006/11/03/ AR2006110301962.html [Accessed 3 Aug. 2015].

Cfids.com, (2004). *About_Dr_Conley Page.* [online] Available at: http://www.cfids.com/ about_dr_conley.html [Accessed 3 Aug. 2015].

Lad, V. (2004). *Strands of eternity.* Albuquerque: Ayurvedic
Press. Lad, V. (2004). *Strands of eternity.* Albuquerque:
Ayurvedic Press.

Mpkb.org, (2004). *Test: C-Reactive Protein (CRP) (MPKB).* [online] Available at: http://mpkb. org/home/tests/crp [Accessed 3 Aug. 2015].

ScienceDaily, (2004). *Images Of Desire: Brain Regions Activated By Food Craving Overlap With Areas Implicated In Drug Craving.* [online] Available at: http://www.sciencedaily. com/releases/2004/11/041108025155.htm [Accessed 3 Aug. 2015].

Binkley, H., Schroyer, T. and Catalfano, J. (2003). Latex Allergies: A Review of Recognition, Evaluation, Management, Prevention, Education, and Alternative Product Use. *Journal of Athletic Training,* [online] 38(2), p.133. Available at: http://www.ncbi.nlm.nih.gov/ pmc/articles/PMC164902/ [Accessed 3 Aug. 2015].

Bodylogicmd.com, (2003). *Hormone Imbalance in Men - Male Hormone Imbalance - Hormone Imbalance in Men - Male Hormone Imbalance.* [online] Available at: https:// www.bodylogicmd.com/for-men/hormone-imbalance-in-men [Accessed 3 Aug. 2015].

Lad, V. (2002). *Textbook of Ayurveda.* Albuquerque, N.M.: Ayurvedic Press
Lad, V. (2002). *Textbook of Ayurveda.* Albuquerque, N.M.: Ayurvedic Press.

Hyman, M. (2010). *How to Stop Attacking Yourself: 9 Steps to Heal Autoimmune Disease.* [online] The Huffington Post. Available at: http://www.huffingtonpost.com/dr-mark- hyman/how-to-stop-attacking-you_b_657395.html [Accessed 3 Aug. 2015].

Noakes, T., Peltonen, J. and Rusko, H. (2001). Evidence that a central governor regulates exercise performance during acute hypoxia and hyperoxia. *Journal of Experimental Biology,* [online] 204(18), pp.3225-3234. Available at: http://jeb.biologists.org/ content/204/18/3225.full [Accessed 3 Aug. 2015].

Lad, V. (1998). *The complete book of Ayurvedic home remedies.* New York: Harmony Books. The Herb Companion Staff, (1998). *Ancient Herbal Remedies.* [online] Mother Earth Living.
Available at: http://www.motherearthliving.com/plant-profile/the-origins-of-herbal-medicines.aspx [Accessed 3 Aug. 2015].

Williams, R. (1998). *Biochemical Individuality: The Key to Understanding What Shapes Your Health.* [online] Anapsid.org. Available at: http://www.anapsid.org/aboutmk/biochem. html [Accessed 3 Aug. 2015].

Lad, U. and Lad, V.(1997). *Ayurvedic cooking for self-healing.* Albuquerque, N.M.: Ayurvedic Press.

Chapter 6
Lad, V. (1996). *Secrets of the pulse.* Albuquerque, NM: Ayurvedic Press.
Lad, V. and Frawley, D. (1986). *The yoga of herbs.* Santa Fe, N.M.: Lotus
Press. Lad, V.(1984). *Ayurveda.* Santa Fe, N.M.: Lotus Press.
Davis, W. (1972). *Money talks - William Davis translates.* London: Deutsch.
Davis, W.(1798). *A complete treatise of land surveying.* London: Printed for the author, and sold by Faulder, Bond Street.
Davis, W. (1795). *To be sold by auction, by Mr. William Davis, on Wednesday, August 26th.*
 1795 at the Cross Keys Inn, High Street, Bridgnorth; ... Sixteen acres of fine wheat. [Bridgnorth.
Davis, W. (1700). *Jesus the crucified man, the eternal Son of God, or, An answer to an anathema or paper of excommunication, of John Wats entituled, Points of doctrine preached & asserted by William Davis.* [Philadelphia]: Printed [by Reinier Jansen] for the author.
Leavitt, M. (2008). *2008 Physical Activity Guidelines for Americans.* [online] U.S. Department of Health and Human Services. Available at: http://www.health.gov/PAGuidelines/pdf/ paguide.pdf [Accessed 3 Aug. 2015].
Hyman, M. (n.d.). *Scientific Exploration 9 Steps to Heal Autoimmune Disease.* [online] Scientificexploration.net. Available at: http://scientificexploration.net/0-12221-9-steps- to-heal-autoimmune-disease.html [Accessed 3 Aug. 2015].
Chopra, D. (n.d.). *10 Ways to Nurture Your Spiritual Life.* [online] chopra.com. Available at: http://www.chopra.com/ccl/10-ways-to-nurture-your-spiritual-life [Accessed 3 Aug. 2015].
 (Emerging Risk Factors Collaboration et al. 2010). The Lancet http://www.thelancet.com/ journals/lancet/article/

INDEX

digestive, 10, 40, 72, 78, 113, 137, 141, 146, 151, 206, 289, 326, 328

digoxin, 71

DNA, 31, 37, 44, 85, 86, 92, 93, 108, 122, 132, 193

Emphysema, 319, 323, 324

ENDOCRINE SYSTEM, 207

Endorphins, 239

Ergotism, 56

Estrogen, 136

eustress, 200, 202, 203, 274

fatigue, 23, 186, 203, 234, 265, 284, 309

fertility, 76, 118, 126

fibromyalgia, 17, 149, 151

Fibromyalgia, 102, 106, 142, 186

FM Wheel Support System, 7

food allergies, 139, 151, 157, 166, 167

Food allergies, 157, 186, 287

Food Intolerance, 156, 157, 163, 166

food preservatives, 16

food sensitivities, 24, 168, 279, 286, 311, 328

Food Sensitivities, 7, 110, 155, 156, 168, 268, 272

food sensitivity, 23

free radical, 98, 118, 132

free radicals, 123, 132, 133

Functional Medicine, 1, 7, 8, 11, 13, 15, 23, 24, 25, 26, 39, 80, 82, 83, 93, 94, 95, 96, 97, 100, 101, 105, 107, 108, 109, 110, 129, 141, 169, 172, 175, 179, 180, 181, 184, 219, 250, 267, 268, 269, 279, 283, 284, 285, 286, 288, 292, 296, 299, 300, 302, 310, 311, 312, 316, 328, 329, 333, 337, 338, 339, 340, 341, 342

Galen, 42, 43, 61

gastritis, 10

GASTROINTESTINAL SYSTEM, 207

genetic hereditary factors, 107

genetics, 14, 84, 108, 277, 295

genetotrophic disease, 89

genomics, 78

Ginkgo biloba, 71

gluten, 81, 136, 145, 148, 161, 164, 165, 166, 272, 280, 281, 286, 320

Gluten Intolerance, 164, 338

GMOs, 138

Grave's, 16, 280

Greeks, 30

gut, 24, 25, 136, 145, 147, 149, 267, 273, 286, 287, 311, 312, 328, 341

Hatch-Waxman Act, 77

Hay Fever, 322

headache, 23, 155, 162

heart disease, 17, 18, 91, 92, 99, 154, 241, 242, 243, 281, 297, 302, 313, 318

Heart disease, 106, 186, 237, 238

heartburn, 23, 207

Herbal medicines, 29

herbalism, 34

herbicides, 27, 191

high blood pressure, 16, 23, 115, 265, 318

Hindu, 34, 36

HINDU, 34

Hippocrates, 41

HIV, 17, 127

Holomovement, 31

homeopathy, 34

homeostasis, 17, 20, 26, 36, 107, 169, 174, 184, 198, 273, 285, 287

Hormone Imbalance, 175, 177, 338, 343

supplements, 121, 124, 128, 174, 213, 278, 312, 317

Testosterone, 136, 301

Thalidomide, 76

therapeutic massage, 34

thyroid, 11, 116, 172, 174, 178, 280, 283, 284, 285, 310, 311, 340

toxicities, 9, 184

Toxicities, 7, 179, 267

toxin, 11, 73, 180, 182, 187, 188

toxins, 15, 27, 107, 132, 141, 142, 146, 147, 148, 149, 179, 180, 182, 183, 184, 186, 187, 188, 189, 190, 192, 193, 197, 269, 275, 277, 286, 293, 295

Tumor necrosis factor, 134

Ukoks, 32

Ulcerative Colitis, 280

vaccination, 47, 324

vaccine, 49, 52, 73

Vata, 36, 37, 38, 39, 40

Vitamin, 7, 86, 90, 92, 110, 111, 112, 118, 119, 120, 121, 122, 123, 124, 125, 126, 127, 267, 268, 271, 301

vitamin deficiency, 23, 308

vitamins, 27, 90, 91, 111, 124, 125, 127, 165, 173, 174, 177, 270, 279, 287, 295, 307

vitamins and minerals, 111

witches, 31, 32, 63, 70, 79

Witches, 32, 33

yoga, 34, 36, 39, 288, 344

Yuroks, 31

58862865R00191

Made in the USA
Columbia, SC
25 May 2019